LIPITOR,® THIEF OF MEMORY

Statin Drugs and the Misguided War On Cholesterol

By
Duane Graveline, M.D.

Introduction by Kilmer S. McCully, M.D.
Foreword by Jay S. Cohen, M.D.

ACKNOWLEDGEMENT

To all my friends and colleagues in the medical, health, nutrition and research professions whose knowledge and guidance have paved the way to writing this book, my gratitude is endless. Your encouragement and advice were essential ingredients to its becoming.

But the most profound encouragement for my bringing the unknown, hidden cognitive side effects of the statin drugs to public attention comes from the letters I have received from thousands of patients, their families or concerned friends, in our country and around the world. Their almost desperate need to understand what had happened or was happening to them and why--especially in the denial or ignorance of these cognitive side effects by their doctors and caregivers--was a powerful incentive. So many have related how learning about my experience with transient global amnesia through my website has helped relieve the stress and anxiety about their sanity. I hope this book fulfills their expectations for even more complete information and guidance on the statin drugs.

Duane Graveline, M.D.

Contents

INTRODUCTION

In *Lipitor,® Thief of Memory, Statin Drugs and the Misguided War On Cholesterol,* Duane Graveline describes the increasing frequency of transient global amnesia and other frightening abnormalities of brain function in users of Lipitor® and other statin drugs. These drugs are commonly prescribed to lower serum cholesterol levels in the hope that vascular disease may be prevented. These increasingly common and potentially severe side effect are a warning that the "war on cholesterol" may have unintended, lasting and tragic complications.

Dr. Graveline's personal experience with transient global amnesia induced by Lipitor is a documented reason for caution in using statin drugs. His experience as an astronaut and test pilot in the US Air Force makes him especially qualified to analyze the hazards of a drug that has the potential for affecting memory and brain function. Imagine the disastrous consequences if such a brain abnormality were to occur in a commercial pilot who has the responsibility for hundreds of lives!

The analysis of the shortcomings of the cholesterol/fat hypothesis concerning the genesis of arteriosclerosis clearly indicates that this theory has outlived its usefulness. Indeed, careful analysis of the data upon which this hypothesis is based has revealed bias, selective use of data, conflict of interest, and other irregularities of science, placing the whole concept of plasma cholesterol control in the realm of myth and pseudoscience. In fact, recent large-scale prospective trials of statin therapy to lower plasma cholesterol have shown no benefit to all-cause mortality, and several studies show that statin therapy slightly increases the incidence of cancer mortality, offsetting the slight improvement in mortality from vascular disease.

In 1968 I was fortunate to have the scientific background that enabled me to understand the significance of rapidly advancing arteriosclerosis in children with different inherited diseases of homocysteine metabolism. In the first formulation of the homocysteine theory of arteriosclerosis, as published in 1969, I suggest that homocysteine damages cells and tissues of arteries not only in children with homocystinuria but also in the general population. Hundreds of subsequent studies in experimental animals, cell cultures and in human populations have proven the validity of the homocysteine theory of arteriosclerosis. According to this theory, deficiencies of the B vitamins (folic acid, vitamin B6 and vitamin B12), caused by destruction through food processing or by decreased absorption lead to elevation of blood homocysteine levels and consequent vascular disease.

In *Lipitor,® Thief of Memory, Statin Drugs and the Misguided War On Cholesterol*, compelling reasons for a new departure from conventional wisdom about blood cholesterol and vascular disease are effectively described. By dietary improvement to increase availability of B vitamins, judicious use of vitamin supplements, elimination of harmful trans fats from the diet, elimination of highly processed foods from the diet, and control of smoking and other proven risk factors, the mortality from vascular disease in susceptible populations can be minimized. This approach promises to help control the leading cause of death in the US without reliance on potentially toxic statin drugs. By adopting this powerful new understanding of the underlying cause of vascular disease, heart disease, stroke, and peripheral arteriosclerosis will become increasingly rare in a healthier population during the 21st century.

Kilmer S. McCully, M.D.
The Homocysteine Revolution (1997) and *The Heart Revolution* (2000)

FOREWORD

When Dr. Duane Graveline sent an e-mail to me in August, 2001, it led to a mutually beneficial relationship. I knew that statin drugs like Lipitor® could cause cognitive, emotional, and memory problems, but I didn't know that they could cause amnesia. On the other hand, Dr. Graveline didn't know that the so-called lowest dose of Lipitor he received, 10 mg, was not so low after all. Based on his cholesterol and LDL levels, 2.5 mg might have been adequate. Thus, Dr. Graveline got 400 percent more medication than he actually required. No wonder he sustained a severe reaction.

It can be difficult to criticize drugs that are beneficial for millions of people. Defenders of Lipitor®, Zocor®, Pravachol®, Mevacor®, and Lescol® immediately point out that statins reduce the risks of heart attacks, strokes and cardiovascular deaths. This is true, and I am not advocating withdrawing or abandoning these drugs. But helping people also means reducing the risks of serious side effects like chronic muscle pain, muscle injury, liver injury, kidney injury, psychological changes, cognitive impairments, and global amnesia.

Unfortunately, while the drug industry sends out 80,000 sales representatives to doctors' offices, fills medical journals with glossy advertising, and underwrites thousands of seminars where doctors are paid to listen to lectures that are really sales pitches for drugs, information about the true risks is hard to find. I receive many reports from patients who develop side effects with medications, and almost every report contains a description of a doctor who is either uninformed or dismissive about obvious side effects.

That's why *Lipitor,® Thief of Memory, Statin Drugs and the Misguided War On Cholesterol,* is an important book. We have to find new ways to get good, objective information to consumers and their doctors. Scientific studies have shown that almost all of the information that doctors receive about drugs comes straight from the pharmaceutical industry. Studies have shown that good, objective information published in medical journals is very slow to get to doctors, if it ever gets to them at all.

The drug industry makes money by developing new, patentable drugs. Even if a natural food or supplement is equally effective, a drug company can't make a big profit from it, so it will push a drug instead. And like all industries, selling its products is based on selling doctors on the superiority and safety of the product. That's why doctors hear so much about statins' effectiveness and so little about their true risks. That's why so many new side effects are missed in early studies, only to be discovered after the drug companies have completed their research, the FDA has approved the drug, and the package insert has already been written. Indeed, a 1998 study published in the *Journal of the American Medical Association* (JAMA) revealed that new, previously unrecognized serious side effects are discovered with 51percent of new drugs after their approval. Twenty percent of drugs ultimately require new, black-box warnings indicating severe or lethal side effects. All of these problems are discovered later, after millions of people have been exposed to the drugs.

So-called *minor side effects* are also commonly overlooked in pre-approval studies, so these side effects aren't listed in package inserts or the *Physicians' Desk Reference* (PDR). This creates real problems because, when people develop these side effects, their doctors check the PDR, don't see the side effect listed, and tell patients that the drug isn't the culprit. Often, this is completely wrong, but many doctors believe the incomplete, often outdated information in the PDR more than they believe their own patients. Such situations, repeated thousands of times every day, erode people's faith in their doctors, the medical system and the safety of our medications.

Even good doctors make these kinds of mistakes. Many doctors don't know that the information in the PDR is often incomplete, inaccurate or outdated. Doctors don't know that the information in package inserts and the PDR is carefully selected by the drug manufacturers and FDA, and a lot of important information about lower, safer, proven-effective doses is omitted. Doctors don't know that side effects reported in studies and case reports in respected medical journals are often not listed in the PDR. Unfortunately, with time pressures greater than ever, most doctors never conduct searches of the medical literature on their own.

This is why so many doctors don't know that Lipitor® and other statins can cause memory loss. This is why they are incredulous when transient global amnesia occurs. This is why they don't know that these problems can suddenly, dangerously, occur after years of taking statins without problems. Many doctors haven't seen the studies showing that after years of using statins without difficulty, 1 in 2,000 people develop nerve injuries that can be severe and permanent. With twenty million Americans taking statins, that's 10,000 people per year.

Dr. Graveline has seen how unaware and, sometimes, uninterested doctors are about the cognitive problems that occur with statins. He has learned, as I have, that patients and other consumers are much more interested in knowing about these issues. Patients, not doctors, take the risks and pay the costs, so they want to know the true risks. This is their right. The American Medical Association's Code of Medical Ethics states: "The patient's right of self-decision can be effectively exercised only if the patient possesses enough information to enable an intelligent choice." This applies to medication therapy as much as to surgery. "Enough information" means being informed about the true risks.

When this right is denied and people develop memory problems with statins, many of them think they've developed Alzheimer's or had a stroke. Others, frustrated, quit treatment. This is unfortunate, because whether statins work by reducing cholesterol or reducing arterial inflammation or some other mechanism, they do help many people. Yet, to use statins properly, doctors and patients need complete information, but they rarely receive it. This book helps fill the gap. It can help you understand the factors involved in cardiovascular risk and what you can do about it. Good health and good medical care rely on good information. *Lipitor,® Thief of Memory, Statin Drugs and the Misguided War On Cholesterol*, can help you attain both.

Jay S. Cohen, M.D.
University of California San Diego, College of Medicine
Over Dose: The Case Against The Drug Companies. Prescription Drugs, Side Effects, and Your Health, 2001

CHAPTER I
Lipitor® Thief of Memory

Try to imagine, if you can, the complete
inability to formulate new memory.

It is frightening to even consider a state of
mind where you are unable to recall an event that
just happened, even though it may have been
extraordinarily important or meaningful to you.
Picture a beautiful smile, a magnificent scene, or
birth of a baby--even a tragic and terrible accident--
disappearing like a tenuous wisp of smoke only
moments after being experienced.

Almost everyone becomes aware at some
point in his or her life of the vagaries of memory,
the reality that recall is not as precise as we would
wish. Few can say with precision what they ate for
breakfast two days ago or their exact words at a
recent meeting but, early on, all of us learned to live
with these minor and inconsequential shortcomings
of recall for that is our nature. We expect precision
from our computers but accept a certain flexibility
of memory in our personal selves. When we say
inability to formulate new memory, I am not
speaking of our common deficiency for recall of
minor events, those routine matters that imprint our
conscious lives only slightly. I am talking about the
complete failure of the imprinting mechanisms.
There can be no recall because there has been no
memory processing. A person afflicted with this
unfortunate problem is like a record with no

grooves, a blank tape, a pristine computer disc with no information saved on it. For this innocent, this newborn babe, every passing moment is a new beginning. The victim has become like Voltaire's Candide--unrehearsed and innocent, welcoming each new day with wonder and anticipation, oblivious to the fact that this scene has greeted his eyes many times previously. The past has lost its meaning for this poor soul. There is no past, only the present and future.

For most of us, amnesia of this type is something we have heard about when someone experiences head trauma, severe electric shock, stroke, certain cases of extensive brain surgery, or secondary to severe chronic alcoholism. These are all common causes of brain damage. In *The Man Who Mistook His Wife for a Hat*, Oliver Sacks[1] writes a classic description of Jimmie G, a patient with post-alcoholic Korsakoff's syndrome, whose memory for recent events failed in 1945, forever locking him into his WW2 Navy life with FDR dead and "Truman at the helm." Although Sacks saw him many times after he was called in to consult in 1975, each meeting was completely novel for the affable, cheerful patient without a memory.

Another relevant case is that of a middle-aged man who had experienced electric shock and then, no longer knowing his wife, had to experience the emotional challenge of cohabiting with a stranger. His memory had permanently regressed more than twenty years. He was never thereafter able to recall their courtship, marriage and early life together.

A third case told of a young woman who required an emergency neurosurgical repair of a ruptured aneurysm in her brain. The procedure left her with permanent lack of memory for her fourth child, her youngest, whose birth had unfortunately occurred during the six-year period of permanent retrograde amnesia that followed the surgery.

The literature is replete with case reports of this type, all of which make fascinating reading but they have only a superficial resemblance to the condition that is the genesis of this book: transient global amnesia (TGA.) This formerly rare condition, this morbidly fascinating end stage of memory dysfunction, in which the inability to formulate new memories as well as a variable loss of old memories occurs, is now known to be associated with the use of statin drugs. With the experience of the past few years we have come to expect statin side effects such as liver damage, muscle pain, nerve damage and heart failure. Even the dreaded and formerly rare rhabdomyolysis -- a condition that occurs when inflammation of the muscle cells is sufficiently severe to cause rupture of the muscle cells and potentially fatal blockage of the kidneys--has come to be expected from statins since the Baycol disaster. But the ever-increasing cognitive side effects from statin drugs are new and completely unexpected by both patient and physician. They strike at who we are, our very essence, for without our memory, what are we?

Transient global amnesia strikes without warning, abruptly depriving one of the ability to formulate new memories. With no record of the past, every new face, thought, conversation or scene is a unique moment, a novel experience transiently entering a mind suddenly emptied of the past. Think of the utter horror of this instant depersonalization, the anxiety, the frustration, the constant query, "What has happened to me?" Think of the concern of family and friends when their loved one has abruptly become a querulous being who can walk and talk but who has suddenly been transformed into a bewildered creature without memory, pathetically attempting to cope with its strange new world.

This devastating world is known as transient global amnesia.

Years ago, when I was a medical student, transient global amnesia was very rare, almost a medical curiosity, and deserving of only a very limited description in most neurology textbooks. Fifty years would go by before I again encountered this obscure affliction, despite the fact that for at least twenty-five years of this time I operated a busy family practice seeing dozens of patients daily. Now, in the past several years, this condition has reached seemingly epidemic proportions in emergency rooms throughout North America and Europe. Emergency room doctors have hauled out their sometimes dusty medical books and looked with wonder from book to patient as they realize they are seeing what, for many, is their first case of transient global amnesia. These confused patients, asking over and over again, "What has happened to me?" or some similar question, are completely unable to remember the doctor's explanation offered only moments before. For every case of this type of temporary amnesia, thousands of cases of lesser forms of memory disturbance such as extreme forgetfulness, disorientation and confusion have also been reported to statin drug researchers. Most of these cases do not make it to the emergency rooms and are, undoubtedly, extensively under reported.

All of these cases are associated with the use of the stronger statin drugs such as Lipitor, ® Mevacor,® and Zocor®. Sometimes symptoms begin within weeks of starting medication. In other cases several years might pass before the onset of symptoms. Frequently they have been associated with muscle pain and tenderness, the much more common statin drug side effects. Although the overwhelming majority of our physicians are very aware of the association of muscle pain with statin drug use, few are aware of the possible effects of statin drugs on cognitive functions. When I first experienced Lipitor-associated amnesia my reaction was surprise, for in my nearly ten years of clinical use of the early statin drugs in my family practice I had never knowingly encountered cognitive dysfunction. Patients, even less aware of this relationship, are reluctant to report amnesia, confusion and altered memory coming on months or even years after statin drugs are started, thinking it is just old age, an inevitable touch of senility or possibly early Alzheimer's disease. When such patients are brought to the doctor's office with these complaints, all too frequently the doctor fails to consider the very real possibility that such side effects might be due to their statin drug, the very drug he had placed them on for health maintenance purposes, the very drugs purported to do so much good for public health.

This was the situation in which I found myself almost three years ago after I had experienced my first episode of Lipitor-related transient global amnesia. The Lipitor had been prescribed six weeks earlier at the time of my annual astronaut physical at Johnson Space Center as part of their primary prevention program for cholesterol control. When I returned from my usual walk in the woods that morning, my wife saw me aimlessly walking about the driveway and yard. When she confronted me, I acted confused and gave no evidence of recognizing her. She reported that I reluctantly accepted cookies and milk but refused to go into our home. I also refused her suggestion to get in the car so we could go to my family doctor. Only after she called the doctor, an old friend of mine, and held the phone to my ear so I could directly hear his strong counsel to get in the car and come to see him did I do so, but only with extreme reluctance. I remembered nothing of the office visit but learned later that my blood sugar was normal at the time and in view of my abnormal mental status, the doctor referred me directly to a consulting neurologist at the nearby hospital.

I seemed to come to my senses somewhat later while in the office of the neurologist, about six hours after my wife had first noted the onset of the condition. The neurological examination was completely normal except for the amnesia. An MRI was ordered and the neurologist made a tentative diagnosis of transient global amnesia, cause unknown. I had been on Lipitor® for six weeks at this time. He saw no relationship and made no recommendations, and shortly thereafter, while still in his office, I felt completely normal. I was even able to drive home but remained totally bewildered by my wife's description during our drive of how I had spent my day. Three days of uncommon anxiety and agitation followed during which time my mind was racing in a futile search for explanations. Hypoglycemia did not seem a tenable diagnosis, especially since my ingestion of the cookies and milk so wisely offered by my patient wife had no apparent effect on the condition. There was no evidence of head trauma.

I then considered the possibility of electric shock, since as a family doctor I was familiar with this possibility. I had even observed individuals whose heads had inadvertently touched the wire of an electric fence. They had fallen down unconscious only to rise several seconds later and continue their walk, completely oblivious to the fact they had been lying on the ground unconscious only moments before. They had reacted with profound disbelief when later told of their predicament. Focusing on this possibility and using my hiking boot imprints in the soft soil as a guide, I desperately searched the path I had taken on my earlier walk. After spending hours on this project I was unable to find a possibly contributory "hot" wire servicing a garden, shed or neighboring camp. I questioned neighbors on either side of our home, asking if they had seen me walking along the street during the time in question. One of them who had been working in his garage replied that I walked by his house and had talked with a local woman who also happened to be walking by at the same time. He said I had a face to face conversation with her.

I remembered none of this but, because of two strange marks on my right temple, I next focused on the possibility that I had been touched there by a "stun" gun. The marks bore a resemblance to the business end of those personal protection electronic gadgets that I had seen advertised in an old U.S. Cavalry catalogue. I imagined myself as having possibly entered the local woman's private "space" with some off-the-wall word or statement and received a "touch" on the right temple in rebuff. Such was my emotional state during this time.

Although I had only intuition to go on, no proof, the doctor in me made me suspect the Lipitor, since it was a new medicine for me and this was a new complaint. I stopped the Lipitor on my own and had no further amnesia episodes for the next year. During that time I questioned perhaps a dozen doctors and pharmacists as to any record of Lipitor amnesia, always with a negative response.

Lipitor was again suggested by my NASA doctors at my next astronaut physical a year later. They had not previously encountered any amnesia side effects from this class of drugs and I agreed to restart at one-half the previous dose, five milligrams daily, which is considered a very modest dose by most physicians.

Six weeks went by and I experienced my second episode of transient global amnesia. During its 12-hour span, I seemed to regress in memory back to my teens, precisely recalling details of my high school years, but with no awareness of ever having been a family doctor, astronaut or book writer. My first amnesia episode the previous year had been one of failure to form new memories only, a condition usually referred to as anterograde amnesia. But this episode was startling because, in addition to the expected and usual anterograde element, I experienced retrograde amnesia for my earlier life, not unlike Oliver Sacks'[2] Jimmie G, or the other two cases mentioned earlier. In this extremely sobering experience with Lipitor-associated transient global amnesia I regressed back to my teens for twelve hours. During that time I had precise recall for high school classmates and events but absolutely no recall for my college years and medical school training, my busy and productive years as a USAF flight surgeon involved with space medicine research, my marriage and four children, my selection by NASA as a scientist astronaut, my twenty years as a busy family doctor or my post-retirement years as a writer with eight books to my credit. To paraphrase Oliver Sacks' unforgettable description of the horrors of amnesia, many decades of richly lived, richly achieved and richly remembered life were annulled and obliterated from my memory. Only after I regained my senses did I realize the hideous implications of the loss I had sustained during those 12 hours of confusion and frustration. According to my wife I had not the slightest recall of medical training or of being a doctor. I doubt I could have responded to treatment requests for a common cold. I knew nothing of my medical practice or of space research. The titles of my books, as precious to me as children, were meaningless and had vanished from my mind.

The same doctors who had treated me the year before made the same diagnosis this time: transient global amnesia, cause unknown. Again they refused to accept any possibility of a Lipitor association, although by now I was finally convinced that Lipitor had caused my problem. But I seemed to be the only one convinced or even suspicious of a relationship. Alone, I remained on a very isolated pinnacle where I became both the soapbox speaker and audience, defending my conclusion. Even my wife was ready to accept that any relationship of my amnesia episodes with Lipitor® was probably coincidental, hinting that the aging process alone does terrible things to the human body. One can hardly argue with that statement but the doctor in me obstinately saw it differently. These were dark days when despite my conviction, an occasional specter of doubt would reach out momentarily, almost subliminally, suggesting the unthinkable: the possibility of underlying brain disease.

Finally, almost in desperation, I sent an e-mail describing my problem to the *People's Pharmacy* column that is syndicated in newspapers throughout the country. The writers of this column impressed me as being very forward thinking and open to unusual concepts. Their response was very positive and they gave me my first good lead by referring me to a statin drug study at UCSD College of Medicine. I felt a tremendous weight lifted from my shoulders when the principal investigator, Dr. Beatrice Golomb, responded that she knew of several cases just like mine. But the real break came a few days later when Joe and Teresa Graedon of *People's Pharmacy* asked me for permission to publish my letter in their column. Of course I said yes and thereby "Let the genie out of the bottle," as Joe Graedon so colorfully reported to me later. Hundreds of case reports from distraught patients and relatives, and even a few doctors, arrived in *People's Pharmacy's* e-mail and in mine. They described a full array of cognitive side effects, from amnesia and severe memory loss to confusion and disorientation, but each had one common thread – all were associated with use of the stronger statin drugs. The one most commonly associated with cognitive side effects was Lipitor, but a few cases were reported from Zocor and Mevacor users as well.

Among the hundreds of case histories we have received, this first one was exceptional. A 70-year-old woman blessed with a wonderfully bright and witty personality presented her story so colorfully that we include it in its entirety. She lives alone, maintaining her colorful flowerbeds and occasionally splitting wood for her stove when there is a nip in the air. Her story begins with the stove:

"The wood was for my Buck Stove fireplace insert, for heating my house because my furnace exploded a few years ago and, while I was trying to decide what to replace it with, helpful friends and a few strangers kept dumping logs in my yard, some of which had to be split to fit the fireplace. Actually I enjoyed having no heating bills for several winters but will have a new furnace next week.

"On 3 September 1999 I started taking 10 mg of Lipitor daily in pill form to lower my elevated cholesterol. Within a short period of time my cholesterol dropped to a much lower level. About five months later, on 27 January 2000, I went outside to split some firewood because there had been snow on the ground for several days and more was predicted within hours. Each day during the severe weather I prepared enough firewood to last about one day and night. I remember explicitly being outside splitting the logs; however, I have no recollection of how much I split, what I did with it once it was split, or when I came back into my house. The telephone rang and I answered it, fully aware that I was talking with a friend but completely unaware that any time had lapsed

between the time I was splitting wood (and totally cognizant of what I was doing) and the time I answered the telephone (and again was totally aware of what I was doing). It's difficult to explain but it's like time had continued without interruption. I would never have suspected that I lost any time had it not been for the unexplainable things I discovered almost immediately upon the return of my mental awareness.

"After answering the telephone, I sat down beside the storm door leading to my porch. Glancing out the door, I was astonished to see split wood scattered helter-skelter all over the porch--far more than I ever intended to split or perhaps could split at my age (69 at that time.) Although I knew I went out to split wood and clearly remembered swinging the sledgehammer, I had never seen that pile of wood; therefore, I "knew" someone else had put it there. That suspicion was reinforced when I noticed strange footprints all over the snow in places I had not walked. I told this to my friend on the telephone and then began to fret on and on about how anyone could have done that without me seeing them when I was right out there all the time! It's obvious to me now and was to my friend then, that I was not being rational but I failed to see any inconsistency in what I was saying to her! I felt fine mentally and physically, was not overly tired and had no inkling that anything unusual had happened except the mystery of the wood, which would surely be solved the next morning when I checked out the footprints and learned who had split the wood and *how they slipped by me and why they didn't let me know they were there. It was almost dark by then, so I had to postpone until the following day my investigation.*

"After hanging up the telephone, I walked into the kitchen and discovered a plate of partially eaten food on the counter top--food I had never seen before! That was really scary! While the wood mystery possibly had a logical explanation, the food was definitely put there by someone else, which meant that someone had been inside my house without my knowledge. Fearing they were still in the house, I searched every room, including the attic and found no further evidence that someone had been inside. Still, my brain could not even consider that I had anything to do with either of these events. The possibility never once entered my mind. And, again, I thought my behavior was normal and rational but I know now that I was somewhat confused and acted a little out of character. For example, I called another friend whose response was, "Do you have any idea what time it is? It's after 11:00 PM and I'm getting worried about you." I convinced her I was fine and that she didn't need to get out of bed and come check on me! And I went to bed wondering why she had worried about me, why I had called her so late when I would never do that to anybody, and still puzzled about the wood and food. For some unexplainable reason, it never once occurred to me to call the police.

'The next morning I hurried into the yard to check out the footprints, hoping I could determine

which direction they came from and, therefore, have a clue as to which neighbor split my wood. They were all very distinct in the snow and very obviously mine! At that instant I realized nobody had been near my house and that my brain had stopped functioning completely for an unknown period of time. Minutes? Hours? I would never know. I tried for days to recall just one tiny thing about the wood, the food, the time I went outside, whether or not I had come in to use the bathroom, if I was inside when the telephone rang or heard it from outside. (I believe the ringing telephone must have brought me back to my senses but I don't recall where I was when I heard it.) Nothing has ever come back.

"It wasn't until 31 January 2000 that I went to the Emergency Room. And it was not the loss of memory that prompted me to go then. That didn't worry me a great deal. I knew it was not a major stroke because I had no paralysis or numbness anywhere. But I feared it might have been a minor stroke and would lead to a major one. I thought of a blood clot, or an artery clogged up with cholesterol or maybe my heart stopped beating for a while and restarted itself! All possibilities were frightening but since I felt so well I was ashamed to go to the doctor and have to tell him nothing was wrong with me! My children all urged me to see a doctor and my nephew, a pediatrician, insisted that I see a neurologist immediately. In the meantime, I had a couple of strange episodes like I had never experienced before. Once, I leaned over to place a log in the fireplace and my face started getting red

and hot. As it grew hotter and hotter my arms and chest began hurting, it was difficult to breathe and I felt like I was dying. Having never died, I have no idea what it feels like but I thought sure that was it! I don't recall how long it lasted but once it ended I dismissed it as just an anxiety reaction to the concern others were expressing over the need for me to see a doctor. An attempt to get an appointment with my personal physician failed because I couldn't get through on the telephone. Later, possibly the following day, as I was washing dishes my face again started getting hot, my arms and chest hurt and breathing became difficult. The feeling that I was dying was overpowering. When that ended I decided to drive to my doctor's office rather than make an appointment. On the way there I encountered a traffic jam in front of the local cafeteria so I stopped there, ate supper and came back home because, by then, I was feeling great!

"On the night of 31 January I went to bed about 9:00 PM--early for me-- and was talking on the telephone with my daughter when suddenly I announced that I had to hang up and get to the hospital! There wasn't time to explain to her that this time I was really dying! For someone that near death, I was able to get cleaned up and dressed, scrape the ice off the windshield of my 1970 car, slip and slide over icy roads all the way to the hospital ER and wait almost three hours to be seen. My chest hurt so much I couldn't sit down so I paced the floor for an hour or so. Then I forced myself to sit down and write a chronological list of

everything that had happened since I went to split wood that day. They kept me in the ER for 16 hours and during that time I was given a brain scan which eliminated stroke, blood clot and anything else that might have caused the loss of memory. The ER doctor told me he wanted a brain scan because I had experienced a "total global amnesia" episode (his words) and that worried him. After getting the results of the scan he reassured me everything was fine with my brain and he had no idea what caused the TGA. He explained that the other symptoms were panic attacks and gave me some pills to prevent them. I never had another attack.

"Later at my nephew's insistence I saw a neurologist who examined me and found nothing that might have caused the TGA episode. Nevertheless, he sent me to an imaging facility to have my carotid arteries checked and they were fine. He dismissed me saying it was just one of those things that happen for no apparent reason and that it "probably would never happen again." You can imagine how NOT relieved I was to hear that verdict.

"On a hunch, I stopped taking Lipitor around the time I experienced the TGA event. However, in September 2000, eight months after the TGA, my doctor became alarmed when my cholesterol again was elevated and put me on Baycol 0.4 mg. I must say, I was not faithful in taking it on a daily basis. Instead I took it intermittently for about four months at which time it was recalled or I quit taking it altogether. She didn't prescribe Lipitor because I

afraid of it even though I had not yet heard
~~ible connection between it and TGA. Then I
People's Pharmacy article and learned
~, e were others, just like me.

"That one TGA event was the first and last
time I have ever experienced a loss of memory of
any significance. I can't always remember where I
left my glasses and often have trouble finding the
"right" word when I need it but I attribute most of
that to living so long and cramming so much info
into my head for all these years."

These reports are still coming in. All have
been reported to the FDA Medwatch program where
they are still in their review process. It has been
nearly three years since my first transient global
amnesia episode, yet most practicing physicians are
still unaware of the cognitive side effect problem
associated with the statin drugs. This information
must be made available to prescribing physicians in
an effective and timely manner. Currently it is all
but completely buried in the Physicians' Desk
Reference's lengthy list of possible side effects,
beyond reach of even the most dedicated physician.
Patients on Lipitor should be encouraged to expect,
and to report, amnesia attacks, failing memory or
increasing confusion. Their statin drug and its
dosage should then be the first thing a doctor thinks
of, not the last.

Though relatively rare as a side effect, the
capricious and unpredictable nature of this memory
theft, one's very essence, places Lipitor in a special
category. To be unable to formulate new memory--

18

for whatever length of time--is a thoroughly shattering experience, even if one appears placid and controlled during the event, for the true horror comes later when the amnesia is over and you learn of the mysterious journey you have taken into a world with no past.

Like most doctors and patients in today's world, I had come to regard cholesterol as my personal enemy. Over the past decade of annual astronaut physicals, my doctors at NASA's Johnson Space center had watched the slow but frustratingly steady climb of my total serum cholesterol. Despite participation in regular exercise and constant, almost obsessive adherence to a fat modified, cholesterol restricted diet, my LDL had reached persistently elevated levels and my HDL was borderline low. The time had come for a more aggressive approach.

This same scenario replays constantly in doctors' offices throughout the world. No one had mentioned the significant contributions of cholesterol to the proper functioning of a human body. Cholesterol was just there in the body, a sort of filler. From its prominent notoriety, everyone knew only that it was a major component of atherosclerotic plaques. But how many of us really appreciated the absolutely vital role of cholesterol in our body? Looking back, as a thoroughly experienced physician, I cannot believe how gullible I was in accepting such a superficial explanation. But with both the American Medical Association and the American Heart Association actively promoting rigid cholesterol control, who was I to doubt?

I well recall that as a graduate of medical school in the year 1955 I was early on exposed to the first rumblings of the low fat/low cholesterol juggernaut. Even today I remember it clearly, reverberating down the halls of Walter Reed Army Hospital where I interned, already aware of its progressive molding of my thoughts. While still trying to absorb the newness of it all, I watched incredulously as my physiologist friend, Dr. Bruno Balke, at the USAF School of Aerospace Medicine, poured canned peaches in his corn flakes and wolfed them down after a three mile run. Dr. Balke was one of the first disciples of the cholesterol-modified diet. We joined hands then, nutritionally, for professionally already our "hands had been joined" by our "seven-day free floating in water'" experiment in 1961. This space-flight-related "man in a tub" experiment captured international publicity and a "Today Show" interview. Soon thereafter the first inklings of the Atkins Diet reached everyone's ears and we laughed at how absurd a liberal-fat, liberal-protein diet seemed to us. We doctors then were marching lockstep to the music of the low- fat, low-cholesterol band, brainwashed to a man by the powers that be.

When the professional zeal for Ancel Keys'[3] low fat, low cholesterol diet became governmental policy in the seventies, most doctors, myself included, danced happily to the tune. We were thoroughly convinced that the policy was right and equally convinced by our pharmaceutical industry, which supposedly always has nothing but the public's best interest at heart, that statin drugs would work safely when diet did not. The use of statin drugs began to mushroom in the late nineties.

When my doctors at NASA determined it was my time for a statin drug, they recommended Lipitor. It was one of the newer, more powerful statin drugs--a class shared by Baycol, Mevacor and Zocor--capable of producing a reduction in total serum cholesterol by as much as 40 percent, and in some cases 100mg/dL reduction within the first few weeks. How could I refuse such effectiveness, supposedly with only minimal side effects? If anyone in the medical or pharmaceutical industry had any concerns about the possible consequences of such impressive and abrupt reductions in the level of my serum cholesterol, they certainly did not advise me of any of them. Statins were so good they should be put in the drinking water was the most prevalent professional opinion.

As a former military flight surgeon, I am keeping a watchful eye on the possible consequences of administrating statin drugs to our flight personnel. Only recently have I learned how much more liberal our medication climate has now become compared to my recollection of my USAF days. If during the medical examination a statin drug is deemed necessary for the control of elevated cholesterol in an otherwise healthy pilot or crewmember, all that is required now are several weeks of 'grounding' initially along with liver function testing at reasonable intervals. No special consideration is being given to the possibility of cognitive side effects because those decision makers within the military do not yet know this information. These cases and hundreds more just like them have been reported to FDA's Medwatch and to the pharmaceutical companies' adverse drug reporting system. To date no action has been taken, even though over two years have passed. "The subject still is being reviewed" is their most recent response, if they bother to reply at all. The public and our prescribing physicians are still largely unaware of this serious consequence of statin drug treatment. Personally, I think statin drugs should be withheld from both military and civilian flight personnel until further study demonstrates their complete safety with regard to brain function.

A loadmaster reports: *"I am a 39 year old loadmaster with flight waiver for taking Lipitor for my cholesterol. For approximately three months I have experienced "short term" memory loss. It has been such a concern to me that I stopped taking Lipitor about three weeks ago. How long can these memory loss effects last?"*

Flight status is a precious thing to these men. In my experience few would 'bait the lion' and jeopardize their flight status by reporting memory alterations to their flight surgeon. This young man's perceptive qualities and decision-making abilities impress me. On his own he did the right thing. His job is a critical one with absolutely no allowance for error. To have reported such symptoms to his flight surgeon almost certainly would have cost him his flight status.

A military flight surgeon reports anecdotal evidence of cognitive difficulties experienced by himself and several jet fighter pilots after taking the statin drug, Zocor. The best way he could describe it was "a huge difference" in his ability to multitask. The fighter pilots described a vague confusion with noticeable memory lapses.

"I would often forget names of people and places to a far more noticeable degree than what I would say are common for me. After initially attributing our problems to being "close to forty," we eventually associated these cognitive difficulties with the use of Zocor and quit on our own."

This is a devilishly delicate problem for all flight personnel but especially for high performance jet pilots who must function at the very top of their capacity. To dare to admit noticeable memory lapses to their flight surgeon is a striking reflection of the close bond tying them together as a team. This is the relationship that all flight surgeons strive for. If, during my own 10 years as USAF flight surgeon, I came even close to the remarkable degree of trust evidenced in this report, I would be very proud.

Belatedly, after first-hand experience of one of the devastating side effects of this too-good-to-be-true miracle drug, I am now asking the question, "Just what is the role of cholesterol in the human body and what happens if the metabolic balance of this substance is upset?"

This is a question to which I believe I have found some reasonable answers, answers that will surprise you. I found that the underlying cause of arteriosclerosis is almost certainly due to factors other than cholesterol, the substance of our national focus for almost 50 years. I present compelling evidence that homocysteine is a major villain, and explain why the past decades of adherence to cholesterol-and fat-restrictive diets appears to have actually compounded the problem.

But the prevalence of rampant arteriosclerosis in our bodies has not diminished; it has actually accelerated, belying the claims that high cholesterol is the cause. Real progress in the war on arteriosclerosis will require a much more comprehensive approach than our present misplaced dependence on potent statin drugs with their growing record of completely unexpected side effects. For some of us, these side effects have been terrifying episodes of transient global amnesia, confusion or disorientation but for too many others those side effects have resulted in permanent disability or death.

In the following chapters I go beyond the alarming appearance of statin drug-induced transient global amnesia as one of the results of the misguided war on cholesterol. My research, begun on statin drugs and naturally expanded to cholesterol, opened other avenues for exploration and consideration in the treatment of arteriosclerosis, the number one killer in this country. As I dug deeper, another disturbing result of the nearly half-century cholesterol-as-villain campaign appeared: the obesity epidemic. The interconnectedness could not be ignored and in the following chapters I'll share with you the many ramifications of the "thief of memory."

CHAPTER II
What is Transient Global Amnesia?

The onset of transient global amnesia is abrupt, without the slightest warning to the patient that a central nervous system catastrophe is about to strike. Suddenly the patient no longer has the ability to formulate new memories, a condition known as anterograde amnesia. Any sensory input during this time will be preserved briefly, if at all, only to disappear completely and forever, as though it never happened. Although consistently aware of their own identities, patients are often perplexed as to their surroundings and the identity of those around them. Characteristically, these patients repetitively question those present about where they are and what is happening but are unable to remember any explanation. To the consternation and ultimate frustration of doctors, nurses and well-meaning companions, they ask the same question, over and over again, sometimes for hours. The following case report is a very typical example of TGA:

"My husband had been taking Zocor for about 6 weeks. One day he got up from bed and couldn't remember what day of the week it was. As the morning progressed, he couldn't remember the month and date. He could not remember how many stocks we had and numerous other things. He nearly drove me crazy asking the same questions over and over. He became very frustrated as he basically has total recall and is known for having a very sharp

mind. He could not understand how I could know the date, etc. and he could not remember at all. I thought he had some kind of stroke so I insisted that he go to the doctor. The doctor admitted him to the hospital and had numerous tests run on him including a CAT scan. A neurological doctor also did some testing. The diagnosis was Transient Global Amnesia. The episode had lasted about eight hours. My husband took himself off Zocor and has been doing great!"

In most of these cases disorientation is profound. Language and social skills are preserved and the ability to focus attention appears normal but, alas, despite the victim's desperate and almost pathetic desire to learn what is happening, nothing seems to register. Fortunately, most are mercifully spared awareness of their memory impairment and preserve a remarkably calm demeanor, cooperating fully with their examiners. Many, but not all, of these patients will have an extensive retrograde component to their amnesia extending back many years in their lives. Gone are memories of friends and relatives, marriages and deaths, positions held and occupations learned.

Attacks of transient global amnesia are thought to be largely benign in nature with cognitive impairment generally resolving after a few hours. Usually the resulting memory gap is only for the duration of the attack but, for some, the gap extends back into the period before the attack and results in a retrograde memory gap as well.

Characteristically, the neurological examination is completely normal except for the amnesia and, after periods of usually less than twelve hours, recovery spontaneously occurs. This restoration of memory takes place quite rapidly, usually within fifteen to thirty minutes after improvement begins until recovery is complete. During this time patients become progressively aware of their emergence from amnesia and, to the profound relief of those around them, their repetitive questioning finally ceases.

The syndrome of transient global amnesia, which usually occurs in otherwise healthy middle-aged or elderly people, was first presented to the medical literature by M. B. Bender[1] in the *Journal of the Hillside Hospital* in 1956. Since that time it has become a well-described condition, although its etiology still remains an enigma.

In another study of 153 cases of transient global amnesia in 1990, the first major review article of TGA, Hodges and Warlow[2] proposed criteria for the definition of this condition. Their criteria have generally been accepted among workers in the field and have proven to be of considerable value in studying this condition. In particular they have helped distinguish transient global amnesia from other conditions such as transient epileptic amnesia and transient ischemic attacks that may closely resemble it. They proposed: (a) Attacks must be witnessed and information be available from a capable observer who was present for most of the attack. Transient global amnesia may well be a vastly under-reported condition because of the lack of an observer. A patient recovering from such an attack has no recall for the event. The only possible clue that something strange has happened might be the patient's awareness of the unusual passage of time. A patient might notice that the sun is now on the other side of the house and he remembers nothing since dawn, or perhaps he comes to his senses driving down a lonely road, lost, and without the slightest recall of how or why he has arrived at that point. In such circumstances most patients would realize that something unusual had transpired and report such happenings to friends and relatives. However, for brief episodes of transient global amnesia without an observer, there might be no clue. Dozens, even hundreds, of such brief attacks, measured in durations of less than an hour, may occur undetected in some cases and lead to gross under-reporting. (b) There must be clear-cut anterograde amnesia during the attack. This must be differentiated from the common confusion of alcoholism or drug effect, or the numbing emotional shock of a severe accident. (c) Clouding of consciousness and loss of personal identity must be absent, and the cognitive impairment limited only to amnesia (that is, no associated speech disorders such as aphasia or apraxia). Individuals with transient global amnesia are surprisingly competent in many respects. They can carry on a conversation and respond appropriately. Anecdotal reporting from observers indicates that routine tasks such as walking or jogging, riding a bicycle or even driving a car appear to be done as usual. One wonders what might transpire in the event there was an associated retrograde element to the amnesia, which included the time period for training for a specific non-routine task such as flying an airplane. If the individual had no recall for taking flight training could he still pilot an aircraft safely to a landing? So far, we have no answers. (d) There should be no accompanying focal neurological symptoms during the attack and no significant neurologic signs afterwards. Such signs would indicate that the attack in question most likely was of epileptic or ischemic origin. (e) Epileptic features must be absent. (f) Attacks must resolve within 24 hours. (g) Patients with recent head injury or active epilepsy (remaining on medication or having had one seizure in the past two years) are excluded.

Precipitating factors, events occurring in the 24 hours prior to the attack that might have contributed to it, are many and varied. Moderate to severe physical exertion often precedes an episode; activities such as dragging a deer carcass out of the woods, heavy digging, felling a tree, and laying concrete. Unusual emotional stresses such as newly reported cancer, a death in the family, news of a severe accident, a lawsuit, and violent family arguments can trigger these reactions. Swimming in cold water is occasionally a factor, and some individuals appear to recognize sexual intercourse as a frequent, and even consistent, trigger. Occasionally, transient global amnesia is seen after routine medical procedures such as venipuncture, minor surgery or application of the Valsalva maneuver, a "grunting" expiration test commonly used to determine cardiovascular responsiveness. Another medical procedure identified as a trigger agent for a growing number of transient global amnesia cases is cerebral angiography. Whether this is due to the patient's sensitivity to the contrast agent used, or whether the perfusing fluid transiently alters brain cell metabolism has not been determined.

High altitude exposure occasionally triggers an attack. Litch and Bishop[3] report two cases of transient global amnesia in healthy climbers at high altitude, which resolved completely with modest descent and left no sequellae. Cerebral edema is occasionally a consequence of high altitude exposure but only rarely are its symptoms those of transient global amnesia.

As to drugs and chemicals, the commonly used sleeping pill, Triazolam®, has been associated with a number of cases of an amnesia syndrome similar to transient global amnesia. This has come to be known as traveler's amnesia and has been reported occasionally with other short acting hypnotics of that class. An outbreak of dinoflagellate toxicity caused a number of cases of memory disturbance and unusual forgetfulness among exposed fishermen who could not remember their destination and got lost while returning to port. They neglected to perform routine safety and maintenance procedures on their boats and could not recall numbers they had previously always known.

The relationship with transient global amnesia was superficial, however, and probably would not have met Hodges and Warlow's diagnostic criteria.

None of these so-called precipitating factors occur with sufficient frequency to cast light on the cause of transient global amnesia. Their varied nature, all contributing to the remarkably consistent pattern of transient global amnesia symptoms, strongly suggests the presence of a final common neurologic pathway triggered by multiple influences.

The advent of the statin drugs has now provided a new contributory factor, one clearly rooted in the biosynthesis of cholesterol and clearly fundamental to neurophysiologic mechanisms. Reported cases of transient global amnesia associated with the stronger statins such as Lipitor do not reflect its true prevalence because so many cases go undiagnosed and misdiagnosed. Whether 1 in 1,000 or 1 in 10,000 cases, the numerical significance of even "rare and uncommon" becomes very real. Millions of patients now taking this class of drugs--particularly Lipitor, which in 2003 is expected to become the first $10 billion drug in history[4]--are at significant side-effect risk, and transient global amnesia is just the tip of the iceberg. For every reported case of transient global amnesia there are hundreds of case reports of impaired memory, disorientation and confusion among an older group of patients that rarely, if ever, get mentioned. All too frequently, this group is willing to accept old age, "senior moments" or incipient senility as the cause, particularly when their physicians are also ignorant about this side effect of the statin drugs.

As to duration and frequency, most patients will have just one attack in their lifetime. Hodges and Warlow reported in their case review of 114 patients that 85 percent reported a single attack only. Fewer than 3 percent had experienced more than two attacks at the time of diagnosis. The shortest attack of transient global amnesia in their group lasted 15 minutes and the longest 12 hours. All of their cases had reliable observers. Quite understandably, in the absence of an observer, short duration attacks are easily missed. Students of this condition readily appreciate this under-reporting bias.

In one incident, repeated almost daily in military flight crew training, a group of people participated in a high-altitude, low pressure chamber test[3] that called for a debriefing after masks-off demonstrations at 25,000 and 35,000 feet to determine whether anyone had experienced side effects from the lack of oxygen. To a man, each participant denied any problem. Then each subject was shown his handwriting trailing off to nothing during his mask-off demonstration, and a video of himself slumping down in his seat, unresponsive and completely unaware of his experience. A different environment and different physiology to be sure, but with the same resultant amnesia and the same missed symptoms.

Repetitive questioning by the victim during an attack of transient global amnesia is an almost universal behavior. Hodges and Warlow reported a 92 percent incidence of this characteristic feature in the 114 cases they reported in 1990. The ability to perform complex manual tasks is often preserved. The ability to drive a car in an apparently normal fashion remains in many of the cases. A number of other more unusual activities observed in patients experiencing an attack included putting together a bicycle, installation of an alternator in a car and making a wooden stool. In one remarkable instance, the patient continued ballroom dancing although he abruptly reverted to very old, familiar dances. The retention of superficially normal appearance and actions is quite characteristic. If one chanced to meet a patient on the street who was in the throes of an attack, one almost certainly would not know it. Many observers report, as their first clue, a peculiar "absent" quality in the eyes of a patient during an attack. Of course, when the repetitive questioning starts, there is no doubt the patient is functioning on a reduced level of awareness.

The family histories of transient global amnesia patients occasionally include a relative who also experienced the condition. However, in most of these instances the reports are of anecdotal quality only and medical record confirmation is lacking. At most, only a 1 or 2 percent familial tendency is proposed. No instance of this condition in identical twins has been reported which is not particularly surprising since the number of positively identified cases since is unrealistically low, about 1,000. The more recent apparent increase in incidence seems to coincide with the widespread use of the statin drugs, especially Lipitor, but the number of misdiagnosed and undiagnosed cases still distort the statistics.

Just as Baycol had a greater association due to its chemical nature with severe rhabdomyolysis, Lipitor seems to have more association with significant cognitive disturbances than its sister drugs, Mevacor and Zocor. It would seem that very subtle differences exist in this group of HMG-CoA reductase inhibitors and they contribute to variations in the incidences of certain physiological side effects. All side effects seem to be shared among the statins but to different degrees.

Because vasospasm, the abrupt contraction of a blood vessel, has been suggested as a possible mechanism for transient global amnesia, a relationship to the well-known vasospastic component of migraine headaches may be present. As any family doctor can tell you, migraine headache sufferers abound in our society. Although tension headaches are marginally more common, every busy medical office has experienced the recurrent demands for pain relief from its migraine headache patients. In most of these sufferers, the common one-sided headache associated with occasionally severe nausea and vomiting is present. Some suffer with the more classic version heralded by various visual disturbances believed to reflect underlying vasospasm. In such patients, wavy lines and other distortion of their visual field usually herald a headache to come. Occasionally a patient will complain of wavy lines so bothersome that reading is impossible, adding that the headache is nothing by comparison. To their surprise and delight, vision can be restored almost immediately with sublingual nitroglycerine, the well-known vasodilator, and the headache process aborts, giving substantial support to an underlying vasospastic diagnosis. A third of Hodges and Warlow's 114 patients had a history of migraine. Unlike TGA, however, migraine usually strikes the young. They reported the peak age of migraine onset in those patients in their twenties, not unlike its presence in the general public, but occasional cases were noted in patients in their sixties and seventies.

In the past two decades the full gamut of imaging techniques has been used on patients with transient global amnesia. Although some have shown evidence of vasospasm in the medial temporal and thalamic areas of the brain--interesting those who study cognitive effects such as memory--this finding is far from consistent and any relationship with migraine headache seems tenuous at best.

A somewhat more commonly observed abnormality is a condition called "focal areas of spreading depression." The word depression is not meant to describe the patient's emotional status, rather it refers to a localized process of loss of normal brain activity. This is accompanied by marked decrease in glucose metabolism and cerebral blood flow. Simply, this is a localized loss of brain cell function in which the brain tissue becomes temporarily inert, akin to having been "removed." Since glucose is the fuel of the brain, cessation of its uptake can be expected to have dire consequences. Some researchers have described spreading depression as a functional "deficiency" akin to surgical removal and have postulated that transient global amnesia may well be caused by it. However, despite continuing research using the very latest technology, the precise mechanism of transient global amnesia remains mysterious.

Permanent retrograde amnesia has been rare because one is ordinarily expected to recover completely from transient global amnesia. One of the Hodges and Warlow diagnostic criteria is complete resolution of symptoms within 24 hours yet they reported a remarkable frequency of 78 percent of patients who had a persistent retrograde gap in memory. The duration of the permanent memory gap was usually brief, with an average duration of 1 hour out of a range of one quarter to 10 hours. Case reports from Lipitor-associated transient global amnesia show an occasional tendency for "flashback" episodes occurring weeks and even months after cessation of the medication, but reports of permanent gaps have been quite rare. Of relevance is a case with a documented severe and apparently permanent impairment of short-term memory processes. I will describe this case in detail later, but this former CEO level executive officer is no longer able to function in his original capacity.

His present cognitive limitations are associated with severe and near fatal rhabdomyolysis.

The prognosis for transient global amnesia cases consistently reports no evidence of increased mortality or morbidity from vascular causes in long-term follow up. This observation argues against such processes as cerebral atherosclerosis or other hemorrhagic or obstructive vascular events as etiologic agents. The results of advanced imaging technology show no evidence to support the progressive development of space occupying growths or tumors as causative factors other than in isolated cases.

Only with respect to the subsequent development of epilepsy did the study of Hodges and Warlow depart from the usual benign prognosis for transient global amnesia. Somewhat surprisingly, they reported a 7 percent incidence of epilepsy in long term follow-up of their patients. In all but two of these cases the time of onset of epilepsy was within one year of their most recent amnesia episode. None of these patients had a history of epilepsy before their first attack of transient global amnesia. They assumed that the presenting transient global amnesia attacks were actually seizures in which epileptic features were mild and masked by the predominant amnesia. These findings were completely unexpected and not identified by routine post attack EEGs. These somewhat sobering findings serve as a reminder that amnesia indistinguishable from TGA may follow complex partial epileptic seizures. The only clue to this small subset of "pure" transient global amnesia cases is that their attacks seem to be both atypically brief and recurrent. For those having both of these features, the likelihood of subsequent development of overt epilepsy is very great and justifies more detailed investigation, close follow-up and even restrictions of certain activities.

The recent introduction of statin drug-associated cases into this growing "pool" of known transient global amnesia events introduces a new factor in the impressive list of apparently unrelated precipitating causes. To sexual activity, severe pain, cold water exposure, strenuous exercise, and cerebral angiography we now have to add statin drug use. At first glance this newcomer in our list of apparent contributors seems to only confuse attempts to define the etiology of transient global amnesia. However, the mechanism of action of statin drugs, that of HMG-CoA reductase inhibition with its subsequent reduction of cholesterol biosynthesis at the cellular level, brings us tantalizingly close to the 'final common pathway' of transient global amnesia, if, indeed, a single pathway exists. The recent identification of cholesterol's vital role in brain activity as described by Pfrieger[5] makes this all the more likely and opens up a fertile area for future study.

Dr. Beatrice Golomb,[6] the principal investigator of the statin study at the University of California San Diego, College of Medicine, has reviewed the diverse nature of statin associated cognitive manifestations in the many hundreds of case reports that have been reported to her. At the time of this writing she has received some 100 cases of amnesia or similar amnestic reactions from which she has selected 30 meeting her rather strict causality criteria for further study (in progress). Symptoms ranged from those of classic transient global amnesia to "spacey," confusion, disorientation and "spotty," to nearly complete memory loss. She found that symptoms of confusion, disorientation and varying degrees of memory loss occurred much more frequently than amnesia.

Wagstaff, et al[7] have recently reported another major review article of statin-associated memory loss. They searched the Medwatch drug surveillance system of the FDA from November 1997 to February 2002, and identified 60 patients reporting memory loss with statin drug use, In about 50 percent of the cases, the patients noted adverse cognitive effects within two months of therapy. Memory loss recurred in four patients who were re-challenged with the same drug. The authors admit that, in the absence of objective memory tests, detection bias is of major concern in interpretation of the results. Their focus was on reported cases of short-term memory loss, and they gave no special attention to other forms of memory impairment such as increased forgetfulness, confusion or disorientation.

Since certain degrees of memory variability and confusion are more or less normal events in our daily lives, we suspect that the under reporting of statin-associated cognitive effects is profound. We are probably seeing just the tip of a very large iceberg, indeed, and one that will only expand if statin drug use continues without side effect safeguards for the patient.

CHAPTER III
The Formation of Memory and Its Transformation in TGA

Nothing is more precious to us than our memory, for without it we cease to be. Everyone we know and have known, everything we do and have done, and even our reasons for anticipating the future depend upon this irreplaceable miracle of life. Tampering with someone's memory is a serious matter, indeed, and when the medications prescribed for a patient go way beyond their intended purpose-- when they pluck on the strings of memory and destroy or distort the contents--the medical community needs to find out how it happened and what went wrong.

Considering memory and wanting to understand the basic mechanism by which learning occurred, Eric Kandel[1] asked himself, "What changes occur to nerve cells when the brain acquires a new habit or change in its behavior?" He knew that down each of our billions of nerve cells electrical signals travel unimpeded until they reach a synapse, the junction between nerve cells. When an electrical signal reaches a synapse, it must transfer to a chemical signal. Kandel likens this to a train passenger catching a ferry across a sea channel, before resuming his rail journey. The analogy is a good one for it shows us that the critical point in the man's journey is the ferry crossing, the synapse, and the junction that must be crossed if his rail journey is to be completed.

Using lowly sea slugs as his experimental subjects Kandel proved, rather convincingly, that at the heart of the synaptic "ferry" lies the ubiquitous molecule, cyclic AMP. This magic substance triggered a cascade of events in the hapless sea-slug's "brain" that gradually permitted it to move its gill covers 'properly' in response to Kandel's puff of air or electrical shock. As Kandel said, "This response hardly qualified as differential calculus but it is learning all the same." Cyclic AMP had initiated a series of gene switching and protein production that modified the very shape and function of the synapses involved in gill cover motion. Clearly the synapse was a lead player in memory formation. Kandel and others rightly inferred that since cyclic AMP was present in all animals, great and small, its role in synaptic modification was likely to be similar higher up the evolutionary chain. That is how nature is--when a chance mutation occurs that really works, nature is likely to capitalize on it. Indeed, cyclic AMP orchestrates the same sort of synaptic modification in man as it did in Kandel's lowly sea slugs except in man the result is occasionally differential calculus.

A result of cyclic AMP's magical cascade is a key protein known as cyclic AMP response binding, CREB, which Tully[2] believes lies at the heart of learning and memory. In his Cold Spring Harbor Laboratory he directed his studies at the prolific and readily available fruit fly, creating such mutant forms as "dunce," "cabbage," "radish," and "turnip," each incapable of learning certain realities of fly life after being deprived of certain of the cyclic AMP cascade products. To show his lack of discrimination, he also created fruit flies with greatly enhanced learning abilities, approaching photographic memory capacity, wherein a single exposure to a stimulus indelibly engraved its memory into the super fly's brain.

Other researchers have subsequently created amnesiac mice by knocking out the CREB protein, and developed mouse "super-learners" by injecting CREB into their brain.[3] As Matt Ridley stated in his impressive book, Genome,[4] "And from mice to men is but an evolutionary hair's breadth."

The volado gene that seems to bind this all together comes next. Bind is the appropriate term to use because many researchers now think that memory may consist primarily of strengthening or tightening the synaptic connections between neurons. In Chile the term volado means something like absent-minded or forgetful and is generally applied to professors. Davis and his colleagues in Houston[5] used it to describe their findings in fly research. Their fly was a different kind of mutant fruit fly, one in which the learning problem is with neither cyclic AMP nor CREB protein, but rather with a vital subunit of synaptic function called alpha-integrin, a sort of biological glue.[6] The gene for this remarkable protein is called volado and its function appears to be, simply, the strengthening of synaptic connections between neurons. Astonishingly, it may be that these synaptic connections between nerve cells not only are the mechanism of memory, they are the memory itself! The implications of this startling statement are profound. and most certainly provide far more questions than answers as to just how this might be accomplished.

And into the mix strolls Pfrieger[7] with his astounding report that yet another substance is vital to synaptic formation--cholesterol. The very substance we have demonized as mankind's worst enemy, an indiscriminate blocker of arteries, the very stuff that pharmaceutical companies have devoted countless billions of research dollars to protect us from, is also our key to learning and memory. Obviously, cholesterol deserved to be re-evaluated and its importance in the body needed to be redefined.

Pfrieger headed two teams of researchers who examined whether neurons can form contacts themselves or whether they need help from so-called glial cells. Glial cells form much of the brain tissue and have long been known to support its development and function. Using cell culture techniques, they found that although neurons can grow under glial-free conditions, few functional synapses are generated. They knew that glial cells produced a powerful factor that greatly potentiates synaptic development but the nature of this synaptogenic factor had eluded researchers for years. Finally they learned its secret--the mystery substance was cholesterol.

Pfreiger's group found that nerve cells must have external sources of cholesterol to form synaptic contacts. The brain cannot tap the cholesterol supply of the blood for this purpose, since the lipoproteins that transport cholesterol are too big to pass the blood-brain barrier. Therefore, brain cells must make their own synthesis of cholesterol and, in this highly specialized organ of the body, the glial cells provide that cholesterol.

Many questions still exist about the precise mechanism by which cholesterol modulates the formation and function of those magic contact points between brain cells known as synapses, but there is no longer the slightest doubt that it is vital to this role and must be present in sufficient quantity. Not bad press for a substance defined over the past decades as so notorious it can now be used to frighten small children about their eating habits.

As to the statin drugs, there is little doubt that any interference with cholesterol biosynthesis at the cellular level is likely to play havoc with synaptic formation and function. Of all the statin drugs currently in use, atorvastatin, lovastatin and simvastatin are much more lipophilic in nature than the others and, thus, are far more capable of crossing the blood-brain barrier and inducing central nervous system disturbances. The others tend to be more hydrophilic and much less likely to affect the brain.[8] Also of relevance here is the observation by Wagstaff, et al,[9] that the overwhelming majority of cognitive adverse drug events reported to Medwatch in their comprehensive review were associated with the more lipophilic statins.

If a spreading depression ever found fertile ground for evolution into full blown transient global amnesia or any other memory dysfunction, it would be in a brain laced with statins and thus capable of only miserly levels of cholesterol biosynthesis. Cholesterol is not only the most abundant organic molecule of our brain, it is the most important. Statin-associated memory dysfunction is grossly under-reported because people do not expect it, and subtle memory impairment is so easily blamed on nature. If getting lost on the highway during the trip to the office, forgetting your social security number, not remembering your investments, or the birthdays of your wife and children for an entire morning can be written off as early senility, what of the far more subtle lapses? How dramatic must these lapses be before they surface into consciousness as something out of character for the average person?

A good analogy to use in explaining the pathways in our bodies for cholesterol biosynthesis and the statin drug mechanism of action is to borrow the plot of the most convoluted spy novel and multiply it by a factor of a thousand. One may then come close to the complex chemical and molecular inter-relationships taking place in every cell of the body. Into these delicate molecular factories throw a strong statin drug capable of some 40 percent reduction in cholesterol biosynthesis, and wipe out a similar percentage of the vital ubiquinones and dolichols as collateral damage. The ubiquinones, the chemical compounds involved in many vital functions of the body, are involved in and indispensable to every cell in our body. The dolichols, a class of compounds severely compromised by the statin drug's HMG-CoA inhibitor effect, assist in the identification and direction of proteins to their proper target in the intracellular activity of the body. Finally, add cholesterol's recently recognized role in synaptic formation and function and then try to predict what is going to happen with any certainty.

The statin drugs are in widespread use today and the trend to promote their use even more broadly seems inevitable at present, particularly when one considers the proliferating TV commercial exposure. One doctor, extremely skeptical that cognitive side effects could be associated with statin drug use, claimed that the only problem with statins lies in the fact that they are not getting to everyone who needs them.

Currently most practicing physicians feel that the statins are the best drugs available for high-risk stroke and heart attack patients and are clearly to be recommended when more conservative measures such as diet and exercise are inadequate. There is no doubt that statin drugs substantially reduce cholesterol levels in most people, but there is growing concern among researchers reporting on major clinical trials that cholesterol reduction is not leading to significant reductions in cardiovascular disease mortality. [10,11,12]

Even when statin therapy does seem to increase survival in CHD patients as reported by Collins, et al, for a large group of diabetics and non-diabetics treated with simvastatin for occlusive arterial disease,[13] one must be wary of the confusing and often misleading use of statistics presented in many randomized controlled trials. For a masterful discussion of the use of statistics to confuse the reader and inflate the true benefit of statin therapy, one need only read Dr. Uffe Ravnskov's book, *The Cholesterol Myths.*[14]

Additionally in his book, Ravnskov reported of the recent PROSPER trial published in Lancet, that statin therapy increased the incidence of cancer deaths , completely offsetting the slight decrease in deaths from cardiovascular disease and further complicating interpretation of reported benefits from statin therapy.

Because of this growing specter of doubt about the effectiveness of statins in the reduction of cardiovascular diseases, and the risks inherent in their use, there is very real concern about the escalating use of these drugs for primary prevention. Despite a diligent search of the literature, one can find remarkably little support for broader use of the statins. Moderate hypercholesterolemics--with or without diabetes, obesity, smoking history, hypertension or a family history of the disease--who are now being placed on statin drugs because "everyone knows they are effective and safe," may be better treated by alternative means.

Doctors must cringe at the rhabdomyolysis deaths, which, incidentally, are still occurring, albeit at a much-reduced rate, but the cognitive side effects strike at our very being, the essence of who we are. The following case touches on this issue of cost versus benefit. It also illustrates that neither relatively young age nor past history of several uneventful years on Lipitor guarantees that cognitive effects will not occur, especially when dosage is adjusted upwards.

"About six weeks ago, my doctor doubled my Lipitor from 20 milligrams to 40 milligrams. For about the past four weeks I have experienced progressive memory loss. I couldn't remember my brother's phone number. I couldn't find my baby's plate of food after preparing it. I couldn't remember recent trips. I couldn't remember to attend a meeting. I couldn't remember a restaurant I ate in and numerous other similar episodes. This is totally out of character for me. I have called my doctor and am awaiting his return call. For your information, I am 39 years old and have been on Lipitor about four years."

Neither the patient nor the doctor currently suspects the possibility that amnesia, memory disturbance, increasing confusion and disorientation can be associated with statin drug use. The case reports that cause us great distress come from the sons and daughters of elderly mothers or fathers in nursing homes who report of their parent's swift slide into dementia shortly after statins were initiated. Their doctors have told them that it was senile dementia or Alzheimer's, but they now strongly suspect a statin component and are angry that the drug was not withdrawn before the parent's death.

Most people in our society are sufficiently realistic to know there is no perfect drug. They understand untoward effects and sensitivity reactions. As Jay Cohen said in his extraordinary book, *Over Dose, The Case Against the Drug Companies*,[15] "Each time an individual takes a new drug, it is the beginning of an experiment." What people don't accept is not being told about the risks involved. In the past three or so years, dozens of amnesia case reports and hundreds, even thousands, of memory dysfunction cases have been reported. Still, inexcusably, neither patients nor their prescribing doctors have yet been made aware of the relationship between the prescriptions they take and the resulting side effects.

CHAPTER IV
How the Statin Drugs Work

The development of statin drugs was an almost inevitable phenomenon. After decades of concentrating on cholesterol as the supposed culprit in arteriosclerosis and atherosclerosis, the pharmaceutical community wasn't about to waste its time and resources looking for anything except the simplest way to "cut it off at the pass."

The biogenesis of cholesterol starts from a simple chemical reaction: Under the influence of ultraviolet radiation, photosynthetic plants combine water with carbon dioxide, the well-known gas we exhale in every breath, to form glucose, the fuel of our bodies.

From this humble origin, the first step toward production of cholesterol in the human body involves the process of glycolosis in which glucose is converted into the two-carbon molecule, building blocks of life known as acetyl-CoA. These simple fragments then combine to start the cholesterol biosynthetic pathway. Next, three molecules of Acetyl-CoA combine stepwise to form the six-carbon hydroxymethyl glutaric acid part of the intermediate complex known as HMG-CoA, which has proven to be the Achilles heel of cholesterol biosynthesis.

This is the weak point in the chain of events the pharmaceutical industry was looking for and the one that enabled them to develop their statin drugs, for when two molecules of HMG-CoA next combined to form the ubiquitous mevalonic acid, the enzyme, HMG-CoA reductase was required. This enzyme was quite easily inhibited and suddenly a multibillion-dollar industry was born with the development of the HMG-CoA reductase inhibitors known as the statin drugs. Whether Lipitor, Mevacor, Zocor, Pravachol, or the ill-fated Baycol, all use the same mechanism and are merely variations of the same theme as marketed by different pharmaceutical companies to obtain market share.

One can imagine the chagrin of the pharmaceutical industry to discover in a simple yeast from the Orient that Mother Nature already had provided her very own "completely natural" HMG- CoA inhibitor, red yeast rice. For thousands of years this yeast, known as *Monascus purpureus*, has been used to ferment rice into wine and as both a spice and preservative.[1] Needless to say, any possible interference of this oriental fermentation product with our emerging statin drug industry was obviated by Merck's patent--the first ever filed on a naturally occurring substance. Mother Nature's cholestin would never compete with Merck's identical product, lovastatin, which has the trade name of Mevacor.

Research biochemists soon identified the HMG-CoA reductase step as a natural control point for cholesterol synthesis since the reaction was not reversible and it was the slowest step of the entire cholesterol pathway. It seemed a natural point for cholesterol control--the pharmaceutical companies now had their "corral." One can almost feel the pulse of industry leaders quicken in anticipation of the potential market size.

Cholesterol, discovered as a major constituent of gallstones, was identified in 1775 as the first known steroid. As a steroid, it is a member of the vast array of natural products known as the terpenoids. Man has used these substances since antiquity as ingredients of flavors, preservatives, perfumes, medicines, narcotics, soaps and pigments. By 1894 the name terpene was derived from research into the manufacture of camphor from turpentine. The relationship of steroids to the terpenoids was not discovered until the late 1950's. Since then the modern study of cholesterol has included some of the most creative and productive scientists of the twentieth century. The biosynthesis of cholesterol was worked out by the biochemists Konrad Bloch, Rudolph Schoenheimer, Fyodor Lynen and many others. Bloch, who received the Nobel Prize in 1964, was Kilmer McCully's professor and mentor at Harvard, helping to guide the promising young biochemist and beginning pathologist along his future path of elucidating homocysteine's role in the etiology of arteriosclerosis. The research on the biosynthesis of cholesterol continues undiminished today. Scientists marvel at the astonishing efficiency and sheer elegance of the steroid biosynthetic pathway. Its complexity is such as to nearly defy human credulity.

The mevalonic acid-HMG-CoA reductase step is but the first step on the long climb to cholesterol synthesis. Many intermediate steps are required before the ultimate goal of cholesterol synthesis is achieved. In at least two of these steps, five carbon units of the enormous steroid class of drugs, destined to be used for other biosynthetic pathways in the human body, are involved. Statin drugs, while curtailing cholesterol biosynthesis, must inevitably inhibit the production of these vital intermediary products. One might say these two simple steps are probably the Achilles heel of the statin drugs, in that the side effects resulting from impaired production of these substances may be intolerable or even harmful to many. The pharmaceutical industry has long been attempting to develop a means by which interference with cholesterol production might be achieved farther along the biosynthetic pathway beyond the point where these vital intermediary product originate but up to now have failed. The inevitability of significant, serious and even lethal side effects has been knowingly accepted. Production of the ubiquinone coenzyme is one of these collaterally damaged areas of great concern since the ramifications are both broad and profound. Biosynthesized in the mitochondria--the tiny powerhouse of the cell that is responsible for cellular respiration and energy--ubiquinone functions as a vital and necessary electron carrier to our ultimate respiratory enzyme, cytochrome oxidase. Because of the extremely high energy demands of the heart, this organ is usually the first to feel statin-associated CoQ10 depletion as cardiomyopathy and congestive heart failure.[2,3]

Dr. Peter Langsjoen, a well-known cardiologist, reported at the Weston A. Price Foundation meeting held in Washington. D.C. in May 2003, on the many cases of statin-associated congestive heart failure[4] encountered in his busy cardiology practice. He has become a strong advocate of CoQ10 supplementation for all his patients on statin drugs, as well as limiting doses or stopping statins.

Ubiquinone in a slightly altered form known as ubiquinol is found in all membranes where it has a vital function in maintaining membrane integrity. Compromise of this important role is thought to be involved both in nerve conduction defects associated with statin drug use and muscle cell breakdown. Dr. David Gaist[5] in a study of 116 patients reported a 16 times greater risk of polyneuropathy among long term statin drug users. This new and very serious side effect of statins should be of special concern to diabetics, many of whom have been prescribed statins because of their high-risk status. All doctors know that a very common outcome of long standing diabetes is peripheral neuropathy. To prescribe statins to these patients because of their special predisposition to heart attack and stroke is a serious decision, a delicate balance of judgment that should be undertaken only after painful soul-searching on the part of the doctor. This is the so-called art of medicine--making the right choice of medicines when considering more than one variable.

This new, sobering information is in addition to the now well-known statin drug associated inflammation of the muscles called myositis and rhabdomyolysis, a condition wherein muscle cells break down and release myoglobin causing secondary blockage of kidney tubules, which may also be based on this loss of membrane integrity. Baycol was removed from the market primarily on the basis of muscle cell damage and breakdown. Unfortunately, many deaths resulted before this corrective action was taken. One of the more tragic case reports from this unfortunate era comes from Steve Sparks,[6] the well-known statin activist. He reports that his father prided himself on doing whatever he could to stay healthy. At the time of being prescribed Baycol, this octogenarian was totally self-supportive, very active in church activities and walked up to 4 miles a day.

He was prescribed Baycol at 0.8 mg on 6 December 2000 for mildly elevated cholesterol and had no other significant medical problems. Within 24 days, he was hospitalized with complete renal failure and a CPK of 150,000. He died 24 January 2001. On 10 August 2001, Steve Sparks filed a class action suit against Bayer and began his current role as statin drug activist, determined that what had happened to his father should never again happen to any patient.

A few days later, Steve appeared on "Good Morning America" with Dr. Sidney Wolfe. Since that time he has constantly searched the medical literature on statins and gained sufficient experience to come to the attention of and work with several distinguished medical professionals in the field. His contributions to the preparation of their material on statin drugs is invaluable. He made the transcript of the entire Baycol trial held in Corpus Christi, Texas, available to many researchers studying statin drug side effects. This document brought to light the consistent observation of canine brain toxicity in the animal experimentation phase of not only Baycol development, but the development of other statins as well. Although the relationship, if any, of these observations to cognitive side effects in humans has not been established, the implications are sobering.

Deaths still occur because all currently used statin drugs share the myositis and potential rhabdomyolysis side effect of Baycol, although to a lesser degree. This continuing problem of rhabdomyolysis due to statin drugs other than Baycol is best exemplified by the following case report on file both with FDA's Medwatch and in Dr. Beatrice Golomb's statin study at the University of California San Diego, College of Medicine:[7]

The CEO of a large company began to take Lipitor in 1998 at the time of an emergency angioplasty. His recovery and subsequent course was unremarkable until the past year when two things happened to make this 54-year old man both the luckiest and unluckiest man to come to my attention. Generalized muscle pain ushered in his bad luck, and the diagnosis was severe rhabdomyolysis manifested by extensive muscle cell breakdown, rising muscle enzyme levels and profound secondary blockage of the kidney tubules by damaged muscle cell debris. Associated with this condition were the loss of respiratory control during sleep and the loss of his ability to express or understand ideas. A physical work-up revealed the usual findings associated with severe rhabdomyolysis muscle cell breakdown but it also included the somewhat surprising presence of a profound loss of short-term memory. "Odd" memory glitches had occurred during the preceding year but he had passed them off as due to lack of concentration. His good luck has been the resourcefulness and support of his wife and family.

He barely survived the rhabdomyolysis and still suffers constant pain and weakness, but his major problem is persistent and probably permanent cognitive impairment. According to his wife, his doctors concur that the damage was somehow caused by Lipitor, a likelihood supported by the failure of extensive testing to show the presence of tumors, stroke or even Alzheimer's. His Lipitor was stopped on 19 January 2002.

The most alarming episode of this man's transient global amnesia occurred in April of 2002, three months after Lipitor was discontinued. He experienced a "flashback" reaction comparable to the one that sometimes occurs months after a drug overdose. On 4 April 2002, as his wife left for work, he volunteered to go to the local store for groceries and, after noting the progressive "greening "of their swimming pool, added he would pick up some chlorine as well. He did the grocery shopping with the aid of his new palm pilot and several cell phone calls to his wife about dinner items for the coming weekend. He then went to the Home Depot to pick up the chlorine and a few other small hardware items. When he parked the car in the Home Depot parking lot he decided to transfer his frozen foods to the trunk before going inside. When he opened the trunk the chlorine and the other items he was planning to buy were sitting there in a Home Depot logo shopping bag. The experience greatly upset him, since he had absolutely no recall of going into Home Depot and buying the items. To add to his befuddlement, when his wife arrived home that evening and checked the receipts, they discovered that the Home Depot chlorine purchase had been made the previous day. No one had been home the previous day when he took out his classic convertible, drove to his errand, and then returned home with absolutely no recollection. He was devastated.

When the reality of his memory impairment became clear, other unusual 'memory' lapses were recalled. One of these odd events had occurred almost a year before stopping Lipitor when, while on an errand, he suddenly realized that he was inexplicably heading north on the freeway far away from, and in the wrong direction for, anything he had intended to do. This episode bothered him but he passed it off as preoccupation.

Another odd event had occurred on 27 December 2001 while they were at their lakeshore camp a few weeks before his life threatening rhabdomyolysis occurred. He had left the house at approximately 4:30 am to do some shore fishing, returning at approximately 8:30 am. When asked if he went fishing he could not recall and was clearly flustered, embarrassed and thoroughly upset over his inability to remember. His wife adds that he must have gone fishing since there is nothing else to do for 40 miles in either direction.

His wife then recalled on 2 January 2002, while he was still on Lipitor, he had called her on his cell phone when she was on her way to work. He wanted to know why he was in the Home Depot parking lot. He was not sure why he was there and was flustered, embarrassed and upset not to know. She also recalled that in November and December of 2001 he started some woodworking projects to be used for gifts. After the projects were completed, he would still go into the garage and find wood components already cut, proof that he had restarted the project several times, evidentially forgetting that he had already completed them.

She recorded additional post-Lipitor observations and realized an episode of aberrant behavior occurred on 22 March 2002 that fit the TGA profile. Her upset husband had called her at work, from their home, and commented that it had been a bad day. He started out in the morning to go to the office and then to the bank and had placed the banking items on the seat of his car. When he arrived back at home he realized that they were still on the seat so he took the car out again to go to the bank. He set out on the freeway and forgot where he was going. He recalled that when he suddenly looked down and discovered that he was nearly out of gas, he pulled off the freeway and filled the tank. However, at that point he had no idea why he had even been on the freeway or where he was going. It frightened him so much that he went straight home and determined not to leave the house again that day. When told about this, his daughter commented she had seen him on the road and waved at him. He had looked right at her face while she was waving but had not responded. He had no memory of seeing her or her very distinctive car and, since his car was equally distinctive, the chance of either of them making a mistake was very small.

Since 4 April 2002, no further transient global amnesia-like episodes have been noted. This formerly successful CEO is now "cognitively impaired" and unable to work, testing below the 1st percentile for short-term memory and cognition. He has been off Lipitor for almost six months with little or no improvement in his short-term memory and his case is one of the rare, reported instances of persistent and possibly permanent cognitive disturbance associated with statin drug use.

Of special interest is the fact that three uneventful years passed before this CEO's Lipitor-associated problems surfaced in the form of his first "memory lapse," and another year was to pass before the dreaded complication of rhabdomyolysis began. This is a sobering observation for those who would seek comfort from the fact that they have been taking a statin drug for a year with no problem. The relationship of this executive's apparently permanent short-term memory loss to the rhabdomyolysis remains to be determined. One would surmise that permanent damage to the memory apparatus must have occurred, particularly to the hippocampal area, yet neurologic studies have failed to demonstrate the lesion--an enigma, it would seem.

Ubiquinone inhibition secondary to the new, stronger class of statin drugs is well known to the pharmaceutical industry, which has toyed with the idea of recommending that supplemental Coenzyme Q10 be used by patients on statins. Although the drug company Merck obtained a patent for the combination of CoQ10 with statins in one prescribed dose, no further action was ever taken on this matter.

This oversight by Merck laid the groundwork for Dr. Sidney Wolfe's petition of 20 August 2001[8] and Dr. Julian Whitaker's 23 May 2002 petition[9] with the Food and Drug Administration (FDA). Dr. Wolfe's petition called for special "black box" warnings to doctors and patients about the life threatening muscle damage of statin drugs, calling attention to the fact that 81 people had died from statin-related rhabdomyolysis since the time the drugs were first marketed in 1987. Dr. Whitaker's petition called on the commissioner of the FDA to change the package insert on all statin drugs and to issue a "black box" warning to consumers of the need to take Coenzyme Q10 (CoQ10) whenever they take a statin drug. Of relevance here is the fact that in Canada the Lipitor warning label is strengthened to include warnings not only about CoQ10 depletion but also includes warnings on the closely related L-carnitine deficiencies.

Perhaps it should be added here that the heart as an organ is just another striated muscle, presumably subject to the same statin-related pathology as the rhabdomyolysis of muscles in general. But the cardiomyopathy of congestive heart failure seems based primarily in the depletion of energy reserves at the mitochondrial level. However, both myopathy in general and cardiomyopathy relate strongly to statin drug depletion of Coenzyme Q10 reserves.

Ubiquinone is also vital to the formation of elastin and collagen formation. Tendon and ligament inflammation and rupture have frequently been reported by statin drug users and it is likely that the mechanism of this predisposition to damage is related to some yet unknown compromise of ubiquonine's role in connective tissue formation.

Science has amassed so much research knowledge that very little remains simple and straightforward, so one ventures cautiously into the murky complexity of another secondary metabolite potentially compromised by statin drug use--that of the dolichols. This is an intricate process of cellular activity that has fascinated researchers for years.[10]

Within each of our cells are miniscule factories of immense complexity. Floating in the cytoplasm is a tubular network of membranes called the endoplasmic reticulum. Proteins manufactured there in response to DNA directives are packaged into transport vesicles (small sacs) that are shuttled across the cytoplasm to the Golgi apparatus. The operation of the Golgi, this marvel of complexity which only recently has begun to reveal its secrets to research scientists, has been likened to that of a post office. Electron microscopy has revealed that its general structure is comparable to a stack of "letters" shaped like hotcakes and bound by a common membrane. It is here that vesicles of proteins are linked with certain sugars, zip-code fashion, and directed to their final destination within and without the cell, and it is here that the dolichols play their unique role. Without dolichols there would be intracellular chaos as various proteins could not be directed to their proper target and would, in effect, be dead-lettered. The post office analogy, though childishly simple, comes very close to describing the Golgi apparatus function as we understand it today.

The following is an excellent example from the many case reports forwarded by those in teaching careers whose livelihood is heavily dependent upon the ability to recall and who, therefore, are particularly sensitive to memory dysfunction. His case reflects very well the resulting intellectual "dead-lettering and chaos" when the memory apparatus fails:

"I, too, had amnesiac experiences on Lipitor. On one occasion I lost an entire day--bewildering! A second time I had a memory blackout, I forgot my social security number, my telephone number, my bank card number, even my birth date--I, a university professor for 30 years who remembered everything. Worried that I had a minor stroke I even saw a neurologist. A test for Alzheimer's was negative. Later, because I had leg and muscle pain on the Lipitor, my family physician changed me to Pravachol. Both the muscle pain and the amnesiac experiences stopped. So physicians need to inform their patients on Lipitor and probably any of the statins, of this serious and upsetting side effect."

This case points out the occasional association of muscle problems and memory disturbances and suggests that patients who experience muscle pain and soreness may be more prone than other statin users to experience memory dysfunction. Cell function research is in its infancy and we will no doubt uncover additional complexities and interrelationships, including the elusive mechanism by which cells actually store and retrieve memory, as we uncover Nature's secrets, one by one.

In the last decade mankind received an incredible research result--the gift of DNA mapping--which introduces wave after wave of astonishing new information promising us the ability to tailor a drug to a patient's specific needs based upon his or her genome. The reality is that this incredible feat is already here and will soon be commonplace. Not only will we be able to predict with complete confidence which of our available drugs are most effective for a patient's specific needs, but we also will be able to choose the drug least likely to have serious side effects. DNAprint Genomics[11] is already offering a service known as Statnome to help better match the statin drug to the patient and this is just the beginning.

Specific DNA printing is in the very near future, but in today's world, with our ability to predict side effects still in an almost primitive state, we allow much too liberal statin drug use. As the zeal for primary prevention by both the pharmaceutical industry and organized medicine serve to promote wider and wider utilization of these powerful drugs, harmful side effects become an immediate concern. The physiological implications of these drugs are profound when based on just what is actually known at this time, but when one adds the reality of our present shallow grasp of physiology at the intracellular level, there is justification for the question, "Do we really know what we are doing?"

CHAPTER V
The Role of Cholesterol in the Human Body

___

There is no doubt that the present notoriety of cholesterol has all but obscured its physiological importance and necessity in our bodies. Cholesterol is not only the most common organic molecule in our brain, it is also distributed intimately throughout our entire body. It is an essential constituent of the membrane surrounding every cell. The presence of cholesterol in this fatty double layer of the cell wall adjusts the fluidity and rigidity of this membrane to the proper value for both cell stability and function.

Additionally, cholesterol is the precursor for a whole class of hormones known as the steroid hormones that are absolutely critical for life as we know it. These hormones determine our sexuality, control the reproductive process, and regulate blood sugar levels and mineral metabolism. This same substance that society has been taught to fear happens to be our sole source for androgen, estrogen and progesterone. Researchers marvel at the remarkable similarity in chemical structure these sex hormones have with each other and with the original cholesterol parent from which they are derived. One might say the glaring family resemblance attests to the mighty power of a methyl group here and a carboxyl group there. The destiny of us all is marvelously controlled by such seemingly minor changes.

This same notorious cholesterol substance is also the parent of a pair of steroid hormones called aldosterone and cortisol.[1] Aldosterone protects the body from excessive loss of sodium and water and is known in scientific circles as a mineralocorticoid. It is absolutely vital for life. Without an adequate supply of aldosterone we would be like an ill-prepared desert traveler destined to die of thirst and dehydration under the glaring rays of a merciless sun as water and salt escape from his body.

Cortisol is known as a glucocorticoid because it helps control blood sugar levels and glucose metabolism, but it also has powerful mineralocorticoid and immune system functions and is fundamentally involved in the biologic response to the stress in our lives.

Both of these vital substances are created in the cortex, the outer shell of the adrenal glands. When the adrenal cortex is destroyed by accident, surgery or disease, death occurs within days unless the patient receives aldosterone and cortisol. Like the sex hormones mentioned above, there can be no aldosterone or cortisol unless an adequate supply of the parent substance, cholesterol, is available. So much of our life is dependent on this remarkable substance.

And where would we be without calcitrol?[2] Another offspring of cholesterol, this remarkable steroid hormone is charged with the responsibility for maintaining the proper level of calcium in our bodies. Like sodium, serum calcium must be maintained by the body within a very narrow range

71

for us to function. Without calcitrol the calcium we ingest would pass through our bowels unclaimed. The calcium in our teeth and bones would diminish rapidly, leading to advanced osteoporosis, skeletal weakness and fractures. Without calcium, nerve transmission to our muscles would fail, resulting in a hyperexcitable state. We have all seen cartoons and movies where a doctor gets an exaggerated knee jerk response while checking a patient's reflexes, a sure sign of low calcium levels. Very low calcium levels result in massive seizures of muscles, incompatible with life, in a condition known as generalized tetany. Such is the power of a simple element like calcium on our bodies if homeostatic levels are violated. Proper levels of serum calcium are also vital for optimum function of our immune systems.

Again, cholesterol is the basis of all these steroid hormones without which life, as we know it, would not be possible. But, by no means is the list of cholesterol's contributions to body function exhausted, for there is another class of cholesterol's steroid offspring without which our metabolic well-being might be in serious jeopardy: the production of bile acids. Secreted by the liver and stored in the gall bladder, bile makes it possible for us to emulsify fats and other nutrients. Without bile, we could not digest and absorb the fats in our diet. In the absence of sufficient bile acids we would all be like those unfortunate souls whose intestinal villi are rudimentary or deficient, which causes them to produce voluminous stools of undigested material while they slowly starve.

The pharmaceutical industry would lead us to believe that rapidly bottoming out our natural cholesterol levels through the use of their highly touted statin drugs is a relatively innocuous process of definite benefit to society. But as we learn more each day of this ubiquitous and unique substance, we must question the veracity of their medical advisors. Cholesterol is perhaps the most important substance in our lives for we could not live without an abundant supply of it in our bodies. Researchers everywhere are learning how extraordinarily complex and often surprising are the pathways that produce and metabolize cholesterol in our bodies. Admittedly, even after decades of study of this remarkable chemical, we still have much to learn.

Pfrieger's announcement on 9 November 2001 about the discovery of the identity of the elusive synaptogenic factor responsible for the development of synapses, the highly specialized contact sites between adjacent neurons in the brain, deserves to be cited again in the context of cholesterol's vast importance to our bodies.[3] Not surprisingly to specialists in the field, the synaptogenic factor was shown to be the notorious substance cholesterol.

The so-called glial cells, the non-nervous or supporting tissue of the brain and spinal cord long suspected of providing certain housekeeping functions, were shown to produce their own supply of cholesterol for the specific purpose of providing nerve cells with this vital synaptic component. As many of you may know, the neuronal synapse of the nervous system is the basis of neurotransmission connecting the brain with the rest of the body. The brain cannot tap the cholesterol supply in the blood because the lipoproteins that carry cholesterol--both LDL and HDL--in the blood are too large to pass the blood-brain barrier.[4] The brain must depend upon its own cholesterol synthesis, which the glial cells provide.

This should be sobering news for those in the pharmaceutical industry developing drugs which interfere with cholesterol synthesis, and that is exactly the mechanism of action of the newer statins. One wonders how anyone knowing the mechanism of brain cholesterol synthesis can seriously challenge the reality of cognitive side effects from statin drug use. The only surprise is that there are not more reported cases of memory impairment, amnesia, confusion and disorientation.

This is heady stuff, indeed, for a substance with such a bad press. When and if the industry finally vindicates cholesterol, it will not be unlike posthumously elevating Al Capone to knighthood.

This discussion of the biological importance of cholesterol would not be complete without a review of recent research information concerning some of the other more sobering implications of excessively low serum cholesterol concentrations in our bodies..

Despite Muldoon's findings of no increase in suicides, accidents and violence in his cholesterol lowering treatment groups,[5] Golomb reported a significant association between low or lowered cholesterol levels and violence across many types of studies.[6] As principal investigator of the National Institutes of Health funded statin study at University of California San Diego, College of Medicine, Dr. Golomb is the recipient of thousands of patient case reports on statin drug side effects.

Whereas Wolozin, et al, reported decreased prevalence of dementia associated with statin drug use,[7] Golomb countered in a letter to the editor of *Archives of Neurology*[8] that the Wolozin data could be taken to support a contrary conclusion--that high cholesterol protects against dementia. Golomb cited her many reports from statin users reporting cognitive loss frequently requiring medical work-ups for Alzheimer's disease and implying that the lowered cholesterol levels in such patients appeared to be a contributing factor.

That low or lowered cholesterol also contributes to aggressive behavior, violence, depression, and mood disturbance has led Kaplan at Yale University's School of Medicine to propose a cholesterol/serotonin hypothesis to explain the relationship.[9, 10, 11,12] Buydens-Branchey reported a strong relationship low plasma levels of cholesterol and relapse in cocaine addicts.[12] Although the authors did not report specifically on the effect of cholesterol lowering medication on their patients, the inference is inescapable that such medication, especially with the statin class of drugs, might seriously aggravate the addiction problem.

As if the preceding were not sufficiently sobering concerning the hazards of low or lowered serum cholesterol, we have the report of Horwich, et al,[14] that low cholesterol is a strong, independent predictor of impaired survival in older heart failure patients. From the work of Peter Langsjoen, we suspect a major contribution of Coenzyme Q10 deficiency in these cases if such patients were on statins, but the authors caution that they did not have data on the patients' medical regimens. They imply, however, that low serum cholesterol is an independent marker of increased mortality in their patient group, suggesting mechanisms other than statin-induced ubiquinone deficiency.

Like many other, if not all, chemical constituents of our bodies, there may well be an ideal level of cholesterol in each of us. Low or lowered cholesterol--below our presumed ideal, "normal" range, DNA-mandated to be different in each of us--seems to be associated with a wide-ranging spectrum of problems from memory impairment, depression, suicide and dementia, to drug addiction relapse, and even with heart failure in our elderly. These observations are thoroughly documented and deserve thoughtful consideration by physicians prescribing statin drugs.

I will present more on cholesterol synthesis in Chapter VI, including the groundbreaking research of Dr. Kilmer McCully.[15] His explanation of the intricate processes by which the body manufactures, regulates and distributes cholesterol and other related substances provides critical new information for patient and doctor.

CHAPTER VI
The Arteriosclerosis, Cholesterol, Homocysteine Connection

No discussion of the cognitive side effects of the statin drugs and the pros and cons of their usage could be considered complete without a consideration of the ultimate reason and justification for their use – arteriosclerosis and its offspring, atherosclerosis - the primary contributors to death and disability in our country. This condition of progressive arterial damage leading to varying degrees of narrowing and even complete obstruction of major arteries is the ultimate justification for today's mammoth expenditure of creative energy and hard cash invested toward its control. If arteriosclerosis did not exist we would not be having this discussion about the cognitive side effects of statin drugs. We must now direct our attention toward the cause of this arteriosclerosis, which has led to the creation today of those "golden drugs" known as the statins.

The vital role of cholesterol in the human body is indisputable. Not only is it a precursor of those hormones that control our very lives but it is absolutely necessary for synapse formation and function, those millions of neural bridges linking all nerve impulses, connecting even our thoughts. As such, it is the very essence of who we are. But the time has come to examine the notorious role cholesterol supposedly plays in arteriosclerosis, heart disease and stroke. New evidence has surfaced that points to nutritional factors other than cholesterol that may really be our major public health enemy and that suggests our 50-year war against cholesterol has been misdirected.

No one has done more or worked harder in the past 35 years to determine the cause of arteriosclerosis than Dr. Kilmer McCully.[1] His persistent, pioneering research has revealed a wealth of knowledge about the process of this disease, our most common cause of premature death. Ignoring the huge tide of contrary medical opinion during that period, he insisted that there was more to the etiology of arteriosclerosis than high serum cholesterol. And he was correct, as this chapter will show. Had the medical research field been receptive to his findings or even willing to consider causes other than cholesterol, the present flood of prescriptions for cholesterol-lowering statin drugs with their devastating side effects might never have occurred.

History tells us that some of the earliest knowledge about arteriosclerosis and its very advanced form, atherosclerosis, came from dissections of the human body done in Renaissance Italy. Credit generally is given to Leonardo da Vinci for the first of these dissections in the 15th century. Abnormalities in arterial walls were found early on and related to social standing, for the most severe abnormalities were found in the wealthy classes of merchants and professionals. In the 19th century Karl Rokitansky compiled a comprehensive handbook of tissue changes he had observed. He suggested that elements of the blood, including blood clots and serum, formed layers on the arterial linings. Over time, a hardened, calcified layer resulted that came to be called arteriosclerosis.[2]

In the late 19th century Rudolph Virchow, who introduced tissue microscopy to the field of pathology, elaborated further on the process of this arterial change. Mucoid degeneration was a term he used to describe the very earliest sign of arterial change. In this condition, a mucoid substance is deposited within the intima, the tissue lining the inside of the artery. Subsequently he noted the accumulation of fatty substances from the blood within this mucoid deposit. He called these raised, swollen area atheromas. This word, from the Greek *athere*, for porridge, reflected the porridge-like appearance of the fatty mucoid substance to Virchow's critical eye. The term atherosclerosis refers to the advanced form of the human disease where multiple plaques of this process are present.

Arteriosclerosis refers to generalized hardening of the arterial walls by a collection of fibrous connective tissue and calcium salts. The two conditions frequently co-exist with atheromatous plaques developing in arteries already lined with sclerotic changes. Virchow suspected an infectious factor when he noted that leukocytes, the cells of infection, occasionally were present in the bases of atheroma plaques.

In the 19th century, little did Virchow know that this work might be relevant to the discovery in the 21st century of the use of C-reactive protein (CRP) as a marker of arteriosclerosis risk. CRP has been known for many years as a non-specific test for inflammation. During my internship at Walter Reed Army Medical Center, the caretaker facility of presidents in 1955, this test was available to us. We knew that elevated CRP was a marker for inflammation of many different types, infectious as well as non-infectious. So it comes as no surprise that the presence of leukocytes of various types in the atherosclerotic plaques suggested infection to many of the early researchers. The apparent truth of the matter is that these kinds of cells are helplessly responding to inflammation in the plaques, inflammation due to the toxic nature of the material within the plaques. An infectious etiology for arteriosclerosis was soon put to rest even though today's infectious disease researchers remain alert to this possibility. Only in the past few decades has the infectious etiology of gastritis and stomach ulcers been revealed. That these conditions are now being successfully treated with courses of antibiotics rather than the sub-total gastrectomies performed 50 years ago weighs heavily on the minds of the medical community.

Like others before him, M.A. Ignatovsky of St. Petersberg, Russia, observed that the patients with the most severe arteriosclerosis tended to come from the older, wealthy class. He was intrigued with this clue that nutritional factor might be playing a role in "hardening of the arteries." He and others suspected that some factor in the privileged upper class diet, which was rich in meats, butter, eggs and milk, might be at work. Not a man to be led astray by the ideas of contemporaries that infection might be a factor, he decided to feed this animal protein-rich diet to his unsuspecting research rabbits. The rabbits developed a condition similar to the arteriosclerosis present in humans. He soon published his findings and announced to the world that a high protein diet clearly was the culprit.

At about this time Ludwig Ashoff, a German pathologist, discovered cholesterol in human atheromas and it was found that the plaques in Ignatovsky's rabbits contained fats and cholesterol. Rabbits studies were continued, this time with the emphasis on cholesterol rather than protein and, not surprisingly, the same type of arterial change occurred. It now had been clearly established that experimental arteriosclerosis and atherosclerosis could be produced in experimental animals by dietary manipulation. For the first time, the cause of "hardening of the arteries" and multiple atheroma could be related to some nutritional origin rather than the vague concepts of infection or inflammation introduced years earlier.

In 1922 a scientist by the name of Dr. Harry Newburgh decided to repeat much of this older work by focusing on meat protein rather than cholesterol, which he doubted, by itself, could be toxic to arteries. Cholesterol was just too ubiquitous in the human body. He systematically exposed experimental rabbits to higher and higher doses of meat protein in their diets, each time demonstrating indisputable arteriosclerotic change. Pleased with his protein toxicity findings, Newburgh next explored individual amino acids (of which protein is composed) thereby demonstrating what Dr. Kilmer McCully, in his book, *The Homocysteine Revolution,* called a "near miss" in medical science because none of Newburgh's animals developed arteriosclerosis. The "miss" was the fact that the amino acid methionine discovered in 1922 and homocysteine, discovered in 1932, were not among the amino acids tested by Newburgh.[3]

These are the only two amino acids which, when fed to experimental animals, will produce the "protein toxicity effect" on their arteries. So goes medical research-- illuminating some pathways, obscuring others.

The medical research community then redirected its attention to cholesterol. The mucoid/fat infiltration of the inner lining of the artery noted centuries earlier began to be termed pathologically as "lipid streaks." Fat-soluble stains proved the presence of fats and cholesterol in these streaks. The cholesterol fat was made easily transportable out of the blood by the action of protein carriers, forming the complexes well known in today's world as the lipoproteins of various types. We now know them as high density (HDL), low density (LDL) and even very low density lipoproteins (VLDL), depending on their chemical characteristics and affinity for various types of fat.

Now enter wandering monocytes from the blood stream whose job, among other things, is to clean up foreign matter. These hungry caretakers ingest the fatty lipoprotein particles to become "foam" cells, the key players in the formation of atherosclerotic plaques.

So far, so good. We seem to be right on track--but are we? Problems arise. First, lipoprotein particles, some known also as the notorious LDL substance, with blood levels "too high" in almost everyone, are innocuous when injected directly into arteries and they are not taken up by cell cultures of macrophages to become foam cells. A macrophage is a generic term for cells, like our monocytes, with the capacity to ingest alien and potentially harmful material. It is part of the body's defense system. If macrophages refuse to ingest something, one can usually infer that the something is harmless and non-threatening. Yet LDL is the substance that, in the animal diet experiments, was carrying fat into the lipid/mucoid streaks to become foam cells. Clearly another factor is involved.

Scientists have looked critically at the cholesterol-fat component of LDL to see what has been missed. They have discovered that cholesterol comes in several different varieties. Some, known as oxycholesterol, contain extra oxygen atoms. Whereas pure cholesterol, free of all traces of oxycholesterol, is innocuous when injected into the arteries of experimental animals. Oxycholesterol, obtained simply by exposing cholesterol to oxygen, becomes toxic and highly effective in producing arteriosclerosis in animals.[4] Inflammation caused by this toxic agent could easily trigger a reaction resulting in elevated CRP. Natural cholesterol is innocuous. Oxycholesterol causes intense inflammation but this is not the end of the story. Our story is just beginning.

Now we must now go back and try to determine the composition of the cholesterol in the original animal feeding experiments to determine the true medical significance of the results. It is easy to be confused by the thrust and parry of medical research and a perception once gained is not easily dislodged, and Ignotovsky's rabbit feeding seemed to provide clear-cut evidence that cholesterol caused arteriosclerosis. Rabbits fed cholesterol got cardiovascular disease and died, so therefore it was the cholesterol. What other interpretation could one make?

Back in the early sixties, when the results of autopsies done on Korean and Vietnam casualties were released, many doctors were astonished to learn that the arteries of these 18 to 22-year old young men were laced with lipid streaks, foam cells and atheromatous plaques. Some even had as much as 40 percent occlusion of major heart arteries.[5] Again, our quite natural reaction was that the cholesterol was the proven enemy of mankind, beginning even at this young age. All of this was very sobering information and the message was easily imprinted in our professional minds.

The country was now about to embark on a three decade long application of the cholesterol/fat approach for the control of heart disease. Powered by ample federal funding, the bandwagon began to roll, carrying politicians, university administrators and directors of health departments and health agencies in its wake. These were the days of the Heart Disease, Cancer and Stroke legislation, which suddenly put universities into the health-care-delivery loop where a major effort was the promotion of cholesterol-control programs at the community levels.

As physicians we began to write more and more prescriptions for cholesterol-lowering drugs. We lectured at service clubs and even to school groups on the benefit of cholesterol control and a fat-restricted diet. Any doctor not marching in this parade was considered academically deficient. Thoroughly endorsed by the medical and pharmaceutical establishments, cholesterol control drugs seemed to be the answer. These early drugs had side effects that were at times serious and even lethal, but the statin drugs were yet to be discovered and we encountered no amnesia, forgetfulness, confusion or disorientation.

Fortunately, not everyone accepted the cholesterol theory. Kilmer McCully, MD, working at Harvard during the late 60s, had been involved in research that suggested a role for factors other than cholesterol and LDL in the etiology of arteriosclerosis, an almost inconceivable thought in those days. His interest was aroused when, as a member of the Harvard human genetics group, he was present when pediatricians presented the story of the death of an eight-year old boy. Suffering from a disease called homocysteinuria, the child had died of a stroke at that tender age.[6]

This rare condition had been discovered only six years earlier by medical investigators in Belfast. In the ensuing years several more cases were identified. In this condition, a genetic error occurs in a liver enzyme known as cystathionine synthase. When this happens, the amino acid, homocysteine, derived from the normal breakdown of protein in the diet, cannot be metabolized by the liver as usual and builds up to toxic levels. The arteries in these cases are abnormal, with hardening and loss of elasticity that greatly increase the tendency for heart attacks and strokes. Not only did McCully focus on this observation, but he also knew of the work of George Spaeth, an ophthalmologist friend, who informed him of the dramatically beneficial effect of vitamin B6 supplementation on some of the homocysteinuria patients he had treated. Spaeth's homocysteinuria patients often suffered from a dislocated lens. He reported his observation to McCully that the excretion of homocysteine in the urine of such patients frequently could be increased dramatically by vitamin B6. Two seeds were planted in Kilmer McCully's receptive mind: the amino acid homocysteine, if elevated, causes a condition remarkably like arteriosclerosis; and a simple vitamin, B6, could lower homocysteine levels. He was elated with this hint that a nutritional factor other than cholesterol might be involved, but his thinking was nothing more than a tiny candle lighting the darkness of research on the disease. He was alone with his concept and his original ideas fell on ears deafened by the roar of the cholesterol juggernaut.

McCully hurried to his laboratory and began to apply his skills as a pathologist to some of the original material from the homocysteinuria case discussed at the genetics meeting. He obtained some paraffin blocks containing tissue from the young boy and a few of the original slides. Soon he was able to confirm that, indeed, the walls of the carotid arteries leading to the brain were severely thickened and damaged by arteriosclerosis, a form of hardening of the arteries. He now knew this disastrous blood vessel disease had caused the stroke that had killed the young boy. He found scattered, widespread changes in virtually all the small arteries of the body..

He found neither cholesterol deposits nor plaques, just the routine calcified sclerosis and narrowing that he had come to associate with arteriosclerosis of the elderly.

Soon he had identified ten more cases of homocysteinuria in children, many of whom had died of blood clots to the brain, heart and kidneys. All showed the hardening of the arteries and loss of elasticity associated with fibrous plaques. An abnormal reactivity of the blood platelets was evident in these patients, which accounted for the tendency toward formation of blood clots. Somehow, the presence of elevated homocysteine in the blood had caused the blood platelets to cluster more readily.

Some time later at another genetics conference, McCully learned of another homocystinuria-like case: a two-month-old baby that had died despite aggressive attempts at therapy. This time, the urine contained both homocysteine and another substance called cystathionine, also related to homocysteine. In the case of this unfortunate baby, its metabolic passageway was deficient in a different enzyme and the conversion would have required vitamin B12. When McCully examined the slides of the baby's arteries he found the same arteriosclerosis changes noted in all the previous cases.

By now one should call McCully a medical detective, for that is what he had become. He admits he had difficulty sleeping for several weeks after this discovery because he knew he was on to something of extreme importance.

Like many scientists before him McCully had doubted the cholesterol hypothesis because cholesterol makes up so much of the human body and is so intimately involved in metabolism and physiology. And cholesterol is a major component of the human brain. How could such a substance be sufficiently toxic to cause arterial damage? It did not make any sense to him. A protein component seemed a much more logical factor and vitamin deficiencies simply could not be discounted. His revolutionary concepts for the cause of arteriosclerosis continued to mature but like so many leaders in strange lands, he had few followers. Driven by the frenzied pharmaceutical industry seeking whatever profitable means possible to control cholesterol, doctors continued to write prescriptions by the thousands. These included many diverse drugs such as niacin, bile acid sequestrants like Questran and the so-called fibric acid derivatives such as Lopid, with mechanisms of action that could only be surmised. The side effects and limited effectiveness of these early cholesterol control drugs were a constant source of frustration-- to both the doctor and patient alike--but in those pre-statin days, the scourges of amnesia, forgetfulness, disorientation and confusion were absent.

Meanwhile it was now 1970 and researchers directed their attention to LDL in its Jekyl and Hyde guise, trying to understand why this innocuous substance behaved so erratically. In one instance it would provoke strong macrophage response leading to foam cell production, and at another time or in another form, its monocyte macrophages caused no pathological response.

McCully thought it likely that the receptor for LDL on the membranes of the endothelial cells lining the arteries was the determining factor and that the "activated" LDL, the process that makes LDL extremely "tasty" to a wandering monocyte, somehow takes place in these same cells. This is the logical point at which oxygen could be added to harmless LDL, converting it into the malevolent oxidized foam cell form with abundant cholesterol deposition and inflammatory reaction that might elevate our non-specific C reactive protein test. The jury is still out on this idea, but research evidence is accumulating.

Strong support for this membrane receptor concept came from the work of Brown and Goldstein[7] in their 1970s studies of familial hypercholesterolemia. They showed that such individuals lacked the proper arterial cell membrane receptor responsible for taking LDL with its cholesterol burden into the cell and processing it. The result was failure to process LDL in the normal fashion, which lead not only to extremely high blood cholesterol levels but also to extensive foam cell and cholesterol deposition, arteriosclerosis, heart disease and, in some cases, stroke.

McCully suggests that "modified" LDL triggers a scavenger receptor response on the endothelial cells lining the artery. This results in abundant LDL take-up and cholesterol deposition and foam cell formation. As the process continues, heavy buildup of cholesterol and other fats occurs in the atheroma plaque. In this scenario, cholesterol appears to be passively transferred to the growing plaque, and it seems reasonable to assume that the higher the serum level of cholesterol, the more cholesterol deposition in the atheroma plaque results.

The next phase of atherosclerosis development comes from an increased tendency for blood clot formation within the arteries. These clots become incorporated within the atheroma, resulting in even greater inflammatory response, connective tissue formation and the deposit of calcium salt crystals. This same type of process can happen to anyone with a bad bruise and clotted blood in the tissues where the occasional deposit of scar tissue and calcium can result in a permanent "lump." The end result of all this is progressive buildup of the atheromatous plaque and narrowing of the orifice of the artery, which limit its ability to carry sufficient oxygenated blood to meet tissue demands.

The final scenario in the process of arteriosclerosis and atheroma evolution involves the blood platelets, those tiny bits of tissue floating about in our blood stream. These platelets have the responsibility for sealing any defects in the delicate tissue, known as endothelium, which lines our blood vessels. As atheroma develops, the overlying endothelium becomes fragile and occasionally tears and, at this point, a substance is released that signals both an inflammatory response and a call for platelets to "seal the breach." The platelets rush to the scene to form a protective patch but, at times, so enthusiastic in their endeavor that they form an unnecessarily large platelet clump. This clump has the unfortunate tendency to break off and enter the circulation as a clot, a frequent cause of heart attacks, strokes and sudden death. This was the scenario of death in our eight-year-old boy with homocysteinuria that first directed McCully along the path of arteriosclerosis research.

McCully lacked enthusiasm for the cholesterol/fat hypothesis prevalent in most of his co-workers. Not only was he drawn by the common sense appeal of his research-proven protein toxicity/vitamin deficiency theory, but he also knew the cholesterol hypothesis was lacking in several major respects. The most glaring deficiency of the then current cholesterol/fat hypothesis, according to McCully, was the fact that "the majority of patients with coronary heart disease, stroke and other forms of arteriosclerotic disease have no evidence of elevated cholesterol or LDL levels."[8]

McCully reported in his 1990 study[9] of 194 consecutive autopsy studies of mostly male veterans of finding only 8 percent of cases with severe arteriosclerosis that had total cholesterol levels greater than 250 mg/dL. He found the average blood cholesterol in the group with the severest disease was 186 mg/dL. This observation, perhaps more than any other, convinced McCully that medical researchers had to look elsewhere. The cholesterol/fat hypothesis provided no answers for this prevalent observation nor did it offer any reasonable explanation for how so ubiquitous a substance as cholesterol, a major and vital component of the human body, could provoke the onset of arteriosclerosis.

According to McCully, perhaps the most important shortcoming of the cholesterol/fat approach is its lack of explanation for the rapid escalation in the incidence of arteriosclerosis, heart disease and stroke during the mid-20th century in America. Detailed studies of the composition of the American diet have failed to reveal a correlation between cholesterol and fat content and the major changes produced by arteriosclerosis during this time period. In general, the fat and cholesterol content of the American diet has changed very little in recent decades.

While we see a decline in deaths from heart disease and stroke due to impressive technological advances over the past several decades, the incidence of arteriosclerosis in its various manifestations continues to rise and remains a disturbing national public health disgrace. Due largely to surgical intervention, we have converted heart disease from an acute illness to a chronic disease, with patients now dying slowly of congestive cardiac failure and other slowly progressive conditions. The slight improvements in arteriosclerosis morbidity and mortality rates not clearly secondary to technological and surgical innovations seem to be primarily attributable to smoking cessation and exercise programs.

In "*Arteriosclerosis Reviews*," McCully suggests the possibility that the FDA's large-scale introduction of supplemental vitamin B-6 into the nation's diet in the early 1960s, implemented mainly via voluntary vitamin and mineral fortification of breakfast cereals, may also be a contributing factor to the decline in morbidity statistics.

Another glaring deficiency of the cholesterol/fat etiology for arteriosclerosis was the observation, mentioned previously, from autopsies done on military casualties of the Korea and Vietnam wars. When one thinks about it, how could the extensive lipid streaks and early arteriosclerosis present in so many of these young men, many still in their teens, be attributable to a cholesterol causation when cholesterol/LDL levels in the young, supremely conditioned group were "rock bottom low?"

Fortunately, Kilmer McCully thought about little else and gradually became ever more confident of his homocysteine/vitamin concept. He remembered his original training at the National Institutes of Health in Bethesda on the subject of amino acids and protein formation in the body. His mentor there, Dr. Giulio Cantoni, had introduced his protege to the almost magical substance, adenosyl methionine, required for the formation of protein and many other reactions in the human body. This enzyme was the key ingredient necessary for conversion of homocysteine to methionine. These two amino acids somehow played a key role in arteriosclerosis, McCully was certain of it, but to work in this field or even think such thoughts was almost heresy in the cholesterol/fat dominated research institutions.

He had few allies during this time. Practicing physicians had a mindset created by decades of cholesterol/fat "brainwashing." The pharmaceutical industry had concentrated for decades on the development of ever more effective cholesterol control drugs. To say the endeavor was lucrative is a masterpiece of understatement. Billions of dollars yearly are involved; the profits are almost shameful in their excess. The bandwagon had turned into a "cash cow" for the pharmaceutical industry and there were no friends for Dr. McCully there. Even the food industry would turn up its nose at a man who threatened their highly profitable, low cholesterol, processed foods and unsaturated oils by suggesting that relatively unprofitable fresh produce and, of all things, vitamin supplementation are healthy substitutes.

Finally, after "baiting the administrative lion for years" by investigating "dark alleys" and despite his 28-year affiliation, McCully's staff appointment ended December 31, 1978. One can only applaud the conviction of this man who, despite this setback, persevered. Gradually, as if to help McCully emerge from his doldrums, the seeds of a homocysteine causation of arteriosclerosis began to germinate and emerge from the research establishment.

Bridget and David Wilcken[10] began to publish their series of papers devoted to the study of homocysteine's role in heart disease. These doctors found that methionine given to patients with established heart disease resulted in large increases in serum homocysteine.

Many other epidemiological studies followed over the next two decades comparing the homocysteine levels of patients with heart disease, stroke, peripheral vascular disease, kidney failure, and even deep vein thrombophlebitis, with the blood homocysteine levels of normal controls. The current result of these studies is a consensus among medical investigators that elevation of blood homocysteine levels is a strong independent risk factor for the development of arteriosclerotic disease.[11]

Another research study of over 1,000 subjects from the Framingham Heart Study showed that the higher the level of blood homocysteine, the greater the degree of narrowing of carotid arteries to the brain.[12] The list of studies vindicating McCully's departure from established research pathways now goes on and on. Clearly, Kilmer McCully was "on to something" back at Harvard when he was denied continued affiliation with their "forward thinking" research institution because "he had failed to prove his theory."

This sad state of affairs brings me to another, equally sad affair: focusing too narrowly on the cholesterol/fat hypothesis. Make no mistake, the juggernaut is still rolling but it is finally slowing down as more and more attention is directed to the glaring deficiencies in its basic tenets, and as the appeal of alternative explanations increase for public health enemy No. 1, arteriosclerosis.

After years of study, the role of cholesterol in atheroma formation must be viewed as a passive one. There is now little doubt that a major cause of arteriosclerosis is homocysteine or some process intimately involved with the methionine/homocysteine metabolic interplay but other factors are likely to be involved. Even McCully will admit that adding together the possible contributions of hereditary predisposition, and even the most pessimistic estimate of dietary deficiencies of folic acid and vitamins B6 and B12 in the general public will not explain more than 40% of cardiovascular disease. Other researchers postulate that trans fats, omega 6, magnesium deficiency, inherent thrombotic tendencies, and even subtle anti-oxidant deficiency, as possible contributing factors. Kauffman wrote an excellent review of this subject in 2000.[13]

A recent study of statin drugs conducted by Dr. Rory Collins of Oxford University in over 20,000 patients in 69 British hospitals exemplifies the direction the pharmaceutical industry would like to go.[14] The patients in the study had established, severe arterial damage and were considered at high risk of heart disease. Although a third of these patients had cholesterol levels that were below the level recommended for statin treatment by US guidelines, they--like others in the study--lowered their risk for heart attack and stroke by a third if they took Zocor, the statin used in the study. Dr. Collins' research team also estimated that statin drug therapy for an additional 10 million high-risk patients could save 50,000 lives a year. Collins adds that an additional 200 million patients worldwide not currently in this high-risk group would benefit from statin treatment.

Present knowledge, however, suggests caution against the tendency for broader use of statin drugs. Despite the glowing benefits of statin therapy reported by Collins, he stands alone in his conclusion as study after study fails to support his findings. The Scandinavian simvastatin survival study, CARE (Cholesterol and Recurrent Events trial), EXCEL, the WOSCOPS (West of Scotland Coronary Prevention trial), and the AFCAPS/TEXCAPS (Air Force/Texas Coronary Atherosclerosis Prevention study) have failed to show significant statin benefit according to cardiovascular disease researcher, Uffe Ravnskov.[14] He postulates that every report of stroke or heart attack risk reduction is effectively neutralized by corresponding increases in all cause mortality or cancer death risks.

"Those people taking statin drugs must be made aware of the cost to benefit relationship," states Dr. Beatrice Golomb.[15]

It deserves to be repeated that, at the time of writing of this book, the possibility that cognitive side effects--such as the amnesia, memory disturbances, disorientation and confusion associated with statin drug use--are rarely considered by patients or their doctors. Much more must be done by our watchdog organization, the FDA, and by the pharmaceutical industry to communicate this fact effectively, particularly in regard to dosage. Statin drug use is not all glamour and risk-free patient benefit as strongly implied in the monumentally effective direct patient advertising of Pfizer and other drug giants. Furthermore, since one of the major underlying causes of arteriosclerosis appears to be some defect in the homocysteine/methionine metabolic process independent of cholesterol, there is a need to redirect and reprioritize the use of statins, especially in view of their unfavorable side effect profile.

Despite the glowing reports in the press, strong evidence exists that cholesterol levels do not matter. Ravnskov[16] summarizes that statin drug therapy is reported to be almost as effective for women as for men, despite the fact that most studies have shown that cholesterol is not a risk factor for women. Additionally, the elderly are protected just as much as younger individuals, although all studies have shown that high cholesterol is only a weak factor for men older than fifty. Another observation mitigating against a cholesterol explanation for statin effectiveness is the consistent finding that strokes are reduced after statin therapy, even though high cholesterol is only a weak risk factor for stroke. Further confounding a possible cholesterol effect mechanism for statins is the fact that they protect regardless of whether the patient's cholesterol is high or low.

Clearly, mechanics other than cholesterol must be invoked to explain statin effectiveness in strokes and heart attacks. As A. Ottoboni, et al[17] discuss, possibilities include smooth muscle migration blockage, platelet inhibition, and suppression of pro-inflammatory thromboxanes. These thromboxanes promote blood clotting, are pro-hypertensive and are damaging to the cardiovascular system. They are formed in the omega-6 arachidonic/prostaglandin pathway. That aspirin has a very similar effect on this pathway probably accounts for the statins being hailed by some as the "new aspirin."[18] Meanwhile, the war against cholesterol by both the food industry and the drug companies continues unabated.

For these reasons cholesterol can no longer be cited as the sole or major cause of any patient's progressive arteriosclerosis any more than can smoking, hypertension, obesity or diabetes. It must be considered just another risk factor deserving attention. All of our present well-intentioned attempts at controlling cholesterol do little for the underlying arteriosclerosis.

There is now a compelling reason for a radical change in our nation's diet and less dependence on pharmaceutical "crutches" and fat-free nutrition. To fight arteriosclerosis one must fight its cause. We need a nutrition and health program directed at homocysteine toxicity, the primary cause of arteriosclerosis, society's greatest public health enemy. Only in this way will we decrease our dependence on the statin class of drugs with their mind-robbing potential. We must insist that transient global amnesia is not an acceptable drug side effect. The present level of gross obesity in America is visible evidence of a national nutrition philosophy that has failed.

CHAPTER VII
The Myth of the Cholesterol/Modified Low-Fat Diet

A major part of our heart attack and stroke prevention efforts these past several decades has been the so-called cholesterol-modified, low-fat diet. During this time our morbidity and mortality from arteriosclerosis has changed little, if at all. True, through high-tech surgical intervention we have accomplished a miracle of restoring blood to threatened or damaged organs, but the prevalence of progressive arterial blockage remains largely unchanged. Apparently we have done nothing to stop or even slow down this dread condition. Our burgeoning statin drug industry now feeds on over twenty million users and still, they say, we are not reaching all the people who should be on it. Some would call this medical progress but *I can only call it failure!*

"If the members of the American medical establishment were to have a collective find-yourself-standing-naked-in-Times-Square-type nightmare, this might be it. They spend 30 years ridiculing Robert Atkins, author of the phenomenally best selling, *Dr. Atkins' New Diet Revolution*,[1] accusing the author of quackery and fraud, only to discover that the unrepentant Atkins was right all along. Or maybe it's this: they find that their very own dietary recommendations--eat less fat and more carbohydrates--are the cause of the rampaging epidemic of obesity in America. Or, just possibly this: they find out both of the above are true." This quote is from Gary Taubes' very perceptive New York Times article, "What If It's All Been a Big Fat Lie?"[2] and who among us, aware of the severity of the weight problems in this country, cannot applaud another avenue of inquiry into its cause?

In 1972, just as the American Medical Association and the American Heart Association started the low cholesterol/ modified fat juggernaut on its fateful advance through the American public, a then little-known doctor by the name of Robert Atkins started his own trajectory, named Diet Revolution. He managed to sell millions of copies of his book by promising that a diet completely contradictory to the medical establishment recommendations was the way to go. He promised the public they would lose weight by eating steak, eggs and butter to their heart's desire because fat was harmless. It was the carbohydrates--the pasta, rice, bagels and sugar--that caused obesity and heart disease, he contended. Atkins popularized his high-fat diet to such an extent that the American Medical Association considered his book and philosophy a threat to public health. Because of AMA pressure, Atkins was forced to defend his diet in congressional hearings.

The thrust of Atkin's diet and of the many similar carbohydrate restrictive diets that followed, of course, was to partake of foodstuffs requiring minimal insulin secretion, thereby tending to stabilize the hunger mechanism.

Since Atkins' debut in 1972, additional best selling diet books including *Protein Power*,[3] *The Zone*,[4] *Sugar Busters*,[5] Kilmer McCully's *The Heart Revolution*,[6] and others have polarized the American public on the subject of weight by recommending minor variations on the low carbohydrate/ liberal fat theme. All of them run contrary to the low cholesterol/low fat theme of organized medicine. The AMA preached that obesity and heart disease are caused by the excessive consumption of fat; the best sellers preached that carbohydrate is the villain and that fat is harmless. Despite the popularity of such books, the impact of organized medicine and the combined effects of our pharmaceutical and food industries have been far greater on the American public, and on all kinds of institutional food.

The result is our present obesity epidemic, our worsening incidence of Type 2 diabetes, and the realization that despite lowering blood cholesterols, our incidence of arteriosclerosis and heart disease differs very little, if at all, from thirty years ago. Some are finally ready to say the low cholesterol/modified fat diet has been an unhappy failure on the part of organized medicine.

Adding to this very real confusion, stirring the pot of conflicting ideology, so to speak, is the rapidly evolving reality that the notorious cholesterol may not be Public Enemy No.1, after all. Kilmer McCully's proposition that arteriosclerosis is largely due to alteration in the homocysteine/methionine metabolic pathways with cholesterol assuming a passive role, at best, is rapidly gaining support. Although the jury still is out on this proposition, it begins to seem very likely that the medical establishment, fifty years ago, may have put all its many prestigious eggs in the wrong basket. If you want to go after arteriosclerosis, place your sights on homocysteine toxicity and nutritional deficiencies, not cholesterol. Isn't it difficult to believe that we really have been this wrong for so long?

Walter Willett, Chairman of the Department of Nutrition at the Harvard School of Public Health in Boston, reports from his comprehensive diet and health study,[7] the largest yet, that his preliminary data clearly contradict the low cholesterol/low fat ideology. In an ABC interview on 21 November 2002, Dr. Willett stated, "The public has been told for many years that fats are bad and carbohydrates are good." This radical departure from current nutritional philosophy literally turns USDA's food pyramid on its head. One can imagine the reaction of tens of thousands of well meaning dietitians and nutritionists to such heresy. To make matters even worse he added, "In fact, we've known for 30 or 40 years that that's not really true." Why, one might ask, was this respected and hallowed institution unable to muscle this information into national policy? Not only has our present nutritional philosophy failed to prevent coronary artery disease and ischemic stroke incidence but it also seems to have contributed directly to our obesity epidemic.

Next door, at Harvard's pediatric obesity clinic, David Ludwig stresses the negative impact of carbohydrates on insulin, blood sugar, fat metabolism and appetite--basic endocrinology apparently not fully appreciated thirty years earlier. To eat more fat-free carbohydrates inevitably leads to hunger and indulgence, then weight gain.

"For a large percentage of the population, low-fat diets are counter-productive," Taubes reports from his interview with the director of obesity research at Harvard's Joslin Diabetes Center. "They have the paradoxical effect of making people gain weight."[8]

How is it possible that a country like ours has arrived at such a point where doctors who can find the time to consider and ponder such matters are beginning to feel uncomfortable and more than a little ashamed?

As Sally Fallon and Mary G. Enig have reported in their perceptive article, "The Mediterranean Diet - Pasta or Pastrami?,"[9] it was Ancel Keys, then visiting professor at Oxford in 1951, who first took note of the apparent benefits of a national diet. He claimed his diet was characterized by abundant plant foods, fresh fruits and grains. As Professor Gino Bergami, Professor of Physiology at the University of Naples, reported to him at the first conference of the United Nation's Food and Agriculture Organization in Rome, "coronary heart disease was no problem in Naples."

Dr. Keys was intrigued with this comment and, shortly thereafter, he and his wife departed from their 1952 unheated apartment and the food rations of England to live for a while in sunny Naples. There, as a team, they studied this classic Italian diet but incorrectly deducing that it was low in fat, especially saturated fat. Serum cholesterol measurements of the local citizens seemed to confirm the apparent benefits. They concluded there was an association between diet, serum cholesterol and coronary heart disease.[10]

As Fallon and Enig reported, at first, Dr. Keys found little support for his revolutionary theories. But he encountered a sympathetic listener in 1952 when he presented his views to a small audience in New York at Mt. Sinai Hospital. Fred Epstein, convinced by Keys' data, began spreading the message "with great effect" over Europe and America. Keys expanded his studies and later, in 1970, published his *Seven Countries Study*,[11] in which it was later found that he had used selective data[12]

After this research was published, the "Keys' diet" became government policy and the darling of both the American Medical Association and the American Heart Association. This was the well documented and perhaps poorly defined origin of America's modified fat/low cholesterol rationale, which dominated scientific thinking and research for the next thirty years. Since that time unfortunate changes have occurred in the so-called Mediterranean diet. The food now served commonly is far from the former Mediterranean pattern. As Fallon and Enig so colorfully describe, "It must be distressing (for Keys) to observe sophisticated Italians feasting on such travesties as pasta Alfredo, veal scaloppini and prosciutto, especially to one who had taken the stringent vows of the diet priesthood." Study after study now finds the so-called Keys Mediterranean diet largely a myth--probably a temporary result of the aftermath of World War II deprivation and half a decade of social conflict but one that became the basis of our low cholesterol/low fat diet.

Once our National Institutes of Health had signed off on the concept, however, the American food industry--suspected by some to be behind the whole thing--quickly joined in with a never-ending parade of reduced fat products to meet the new recommendations. The fat content, which to a great extent gives processed food much of its flavor, was eliminated from many cookies and chips, ice cream, milk, cheese and yogurt and replaced by carbohydrates. These carbohydrates were inevitably the refined variety, relying heavily on refined sugar or starch, which, though adding bulk and perhaps taste, resulted in the public eating almost pure sugar, metabolically speaking. Aided and abetted by the missionary zeal of well-intentioned dietitians, health organizations, consumer groups and even cookbook writers, one could almost see America's waistlines expanding.

The impact of low fat/high carbohydrate diets on serum triglycerides was and is potentially lethal. By the late 1960s, triglyceride levels were already rising, protective HDL levels were falling and Type

2 diabetes was doing what it had to do--progressively rise. Endocrinologists like Gerry Reaven at Stanford University could see it happening. They even had a name for it--Syndrome X--but their voices could barely be heard over the roar of the low-cholesterol/reduced-fat avalanche.

And in the midst of all this "low cholesterol hoopla," drugs designed for the purpose of lowering cholesterol were to become the darlings of the pharmaceutical industry. Potentially, millions, then billions, of dollars of profit were to be made. Finally red yeast rice, originally from the Orient where it had been used for centuries as a dietary supplement, came to the attention of the drug industry. They soon deduced that red yeast rice contained a naturally occurring HMG- CoA reductase inhibitor. This was Mother Nature's own statin drug--and the race was on.

Those same drug company researchers soon devised more and more effective statin drugs. In time, the truly effective ones--Baycol, Lipitor, Lescol, Pravachol, Mevacor, and Zocor--were developed, some capable of as much as a 40 percent reduction of LDL cholesterol in just a matter of weeks. Then, almost inevitably, the truly remarkable, even lethal, side effects began to emerge in a public lulled into complacency by ultra-positive direct-to-patient advertising.

The FDA prudently but somewhat belatedly "rushed" Baycol off the market after two years because of dozens of rhabdomyolysis deaths. Rhabdomyolysis deaths are still occurring, albeit at a much reduced rate, but now the issue of cognitive impairment among users of Lipitor, Zocor and Mevacor is reaching public consciousness. All of this for the purpose of lowering the blood level of the substance, cholesterol, that was already known to be absolutely vital for the human body to function. Even our very thought processes demand adequate supplies of this ubiquitous substance. And all of this pharmaceutical legerdemain is being done to control this wonder substance--which only occasionally winds up in atheroma because of misdirected "oxidized" lipoprotein--and which has no demonstrable causative role in arteriosclerosis.

After fifty years of the low cholesterol/low fat diet we now are a nation of fattened sheep conditioned to the erroneous belief that cholesterol is our enemy and almost any food with low or no fat is our friend. Predictably, the natural evolution of all this well-intentioned mind control on the part of the American Heart Association and a host of other contributory agencies has been a greatly increased consumption of carbohydrates by the American public. Being human, we flocked to the tastiest and most readily available source with the longest shelf-life, the refined carbohydrates, which brings us up to date: the current epidemic of obesity and diabetes, but accompanied by largely unchanged serum cholesterols. The ultimate effect of our present sky-high incidence of these two diseases is a population at much greater risk for coronary heart disease and stroke, two of the primary conditions for which the diet was originally concocted to help prevent.

The most basic tenet of medicine, taught to every freshman medical student and reinforced almost daily throughout his training is "First, do no harm." But doctors are only human and they marched with their colleagues, hand in hand, behind the banner of the low cholesterol/low fat diet. That clinical evidence now indicates physicians might have been wrong is undoubtedly a sore point that is difficult for many of them to reconcile. Almost every day a doctor finds himself/herself in the position of making extremely critical, potentially life and death medical decisions, and to have been wrong in health care delivery is not a situation that any doctor can take lightly.

Every seasoned doctor has occasion to recall some of the basic concepts of diagnosis and treatment taught to him or her as a medical student that, in today's world, are no longer valid. Now it seems that the rock solid foundation of the American Diabetes Association diabetic diet may be crumbling. On the one hand, doctors were taught in biochemistry that consumption of fat and protein placed minimal demands on the pancreas for insulin production, yet the standard diabetic diet they were told to prescribe for their patients had a surprisingly ample component of carbohydrates in the form of bread, potatoes and rice. All of these, of course, place heavy demands on insulin secretion. A natural inclination for many young doctors during those early years of medical training was to recommend a carbohydrate restrictive, liberal fat/protein diet for their diabetic patients, but such deviant behavior was not encouraged. Now we find a growing trend among diabetes specialists to restrict carbohydrates in their patients' diet, and it works.

By the time of graduation, most physicians are well trained to walk in step with all their medical colleagues; challenging authority does not come easily. Yet for a doctor like McCully, challenging the status quo motivated his success in his search for the cause of a killer disease. Many doctors are now challenging the national trend for excessively liberal statin drug use. It may be that modest levels of cholesterol are best treated by "benign neglect" or diet alone and the ideal diet seems to be one with more liberal protein and fat, with restriction of refined or all carbohydrates. More aggressive measures to lower cholesterol levels with statins are justified only for those patients in a high-risk category.

The physiologic basis for the carbohydrate restrictive diet has to do with the "Glycemic Index" of various foodstuffs.[13] By eating those foods that have a minimal impact on your blood glucose levels, you will be eating very close to an ideal diet for health. You may still crave an occasional hot fudge sundae and quite possibly should indulge yourself, but select your usual intake of foods from those having a low glycemic index, i.e., those having a relatively low impact on insulin release.

As you review these diets you will observe how very basic they are, even primitive, for to eat in this manner is to regress, nutritionally speaking, 10,000 years to the time before our encounter with agriculture and the preponderance of carbohydrate in our diet. We humans think of ourselves as highly evolved, the epitome of the evolutionary process. We do not easily take to the concept of dietary regression. Thus, 10,000 years ago we did not have a McDonald's around every corner and our blood sugar behaving like a yo-yo. We tended to burn fat and protein. As cave men, we were on a "ketosis high," eating only when we could, not when we wanted to. Our primary fuel was our blood ketones, derived from burning body fat as energy. Atkins liked to say ketosis was so energizing it was better than sex. One imagines the cave men and women had more sense than that or we would not be here. Richard Veech, a National Institutes of Health (NIH) researcher who studied medicine at Harvard before getting his doctorate at Oxford University, was quoted by Taubes in his interview[14] as calling ketones "magic," showing that the heart and brain run 25 percent more efficiently on ketones than on blood sugar.

Researchers finally decided that the carbohydrate restrictive diets are sufficiently interesting to be tested scientifically and compared with The American Heart Association's traditional low cholesterol/modified fat diet. Five of these studies are in progress, none of which has been financed by the NIH. Preliminary results are remarkably similar: Cholesterol levels have improved similarly on both diets, while triglyceride (TG) levels are predictably lower on the carbohydrate restrictive diet. Because present research leads to the conclusion that total serum cholesterol no longer has the same relevance as an indicator for cardiovascular disease, one can justifiably question the importance on any rise or fall of these values. However, the TG/HDL ratio is now felt to have some merit as an indicator for risk for cardiovascular disease, along with the now conventional homocysteine level and, perhaps, C-reactive Protein (CRP). These diet studies do assure us, however, that carbohydrate restrictive diets have promise, not only to curtail our present obesity and type 2 diabetes epidemics but also to enhance nutrition in general and thereby favorably impact cardiovascular disease as well.

Taubes reports that Albert Stunkard, professor of Psychiatry and founder of the Weight and Eating Disorders Program at University of Pennsylvania's School of Medicine, used this concept to treat obesity for fifty years and commented on the results: "I think when this stuff gets to be recognized, it's going to shake up a lot of thinking about obesity and metabolism."[14]

And the process of shaking up the thinking has begun. It arrived--to paraphrase my earlier statement--with the understanding that cholesterol is not the cause of our present diabetes or obesity epidemic, any more than it is the culprit in progressive arteriosclerosis. Clearly, the true cause of this epidemic is a half century of misguided zeal in attempting to control cholesterol through excessive utilization of mostly refined carbohydrates. This failure, in turn, has lead to our present burgeoning dependence on statin drugs for cholesterol control and the resultant "hidden epidemic" of the side effects - amnesia, forgetfulness, confusion and disorientation - from those drugs.

CHAPTER VIII
What Diet, Then? Reshuffling the Food Pyramid

If the low fat, low cholesterol, all too liberal refined carbohydrate diet of the past 40 years has failed, leaving statin drug use and vascular surgery of one type or another at an all time high, where do we turn? What do we do? Our past leaders seem to have failed us. Who, then, is qualified to take the lead?

Dr. Kilmer McCully's far-reaching conclusion--that elevated homocysteine, not cholesterol, is the genesis of arteriosclerosis--naturally led him to re-examine every facet of the prevailing public food habits. In regard to the FDA's diet guidelines, he unequivocally states:

"The Food Pyramid is wrong on two counts: First, it is based on the false premise that cholesterol and saturated fats are the underlying cause of coronary heart disease. Second, it erroneously implies that all carbohydrates - whether refined or from whole food - are preferable to fats."[1]

One has but to look on the bookshelves of the local library and nutrition stores to observe that McCully is hardly alone in his philosophy. There are now many readable and informative books dealing with the subject of how our past decades of diet and nutrition standards have failed us. They very capably present the novel carbohydrate restrictive diet that McCully knew had to replace the old, national diet of the past. The first of these

117

renegade leaders to gain notoriety is Dr. Robert C. Atkins but he was hardly the first to observe the problems inherent in the excessive reliance on carbohydrates in one's diet.

In 1862, the famous Dr. William Harvey imposed the then radical carbohydrate restrictive diet on his obese patient and friend, William Banting. an overweight London cabinet maker and undertaker to royalty, after diet and exercise failed to help with Banting's problem. The regimen was so successful that in 1864 Banting published a booklet, "A Letter on Corpulence Addressed to the Public," extolling its virtues. The booklet sold over 60,000 copies and his diet became as widely know and controversial in Britain (and later America) as the Atkins one is in our century. Banting maintained a normal weight on his low carbohydrate diet until his death at 81.[2]

Atkins, a young cardiologist is 1963, found that for him a low carbohydrate diet worked to assuage his hunger and control his tendency to gain weight. He went on to write his famous book, now in its third edition, on the protein augmented, carbohydrate restrictive diet.[3]

Atkins has been followed by legions of other writers rebelling against the guidelines and even the dictates of organized medicine represented by the United States Department of Agriculture (USDA), the American Diabetes Association (AbdA), the U.S. Food and Drug Administration (FDA), the National Cholesterol Education Program (NCEP), the National Heart, Lung and Blood Institute

(NHLBI), and the Canadian Food Inspection Agency (CFIA). The millions of book sales these various authors have racked up against such odds reflect the awareness of the general public that all is not well with our food industry and national nutrition policies.

Joel Kauffman recently reviewed 12 of these popular books, comparing their strengths and weaknesses.[4] Kauffman describes the two books of this group which do not contain menus or recipes, one by Braly and Hoggan,[5] and one by Ottoboni and Ottoboni [6] as both excellent and complementary. He describes the homocysteine and oxycholesterol portions of the McCully and McCully [7] book as excellent and complementary to the foregoing ones. He praises a book by Berstein[8] as being in a class by itself and must reading for diagnosed diabetics. For people not sure of which diet-based affliction they have, Kauffman encourages a book by Smith.[9] For overweight people who want minimal reading and a simple diet plan to follow, the Allan and Lutz[10] or Groves[11] books are recommended. The Eades and Eades[12] and Atkins[13] books are for those seeking more information and diet plans. Kauffman even considers the special dietary concerns of those from eastern Europe when he guides readers to a book by Kwasniewski and Chylinski.[14] In light of present knowledge, any one of these diets, if reasonably followed, will result in a general level of nutrition far superior to any served up by the low cholesterol, low fat doctrine during our past 50 years of homage.

And the slowly turning tide back to the natural fats that were the foundation of the American diet before the "prudent diet" became the national one is discussed in a paper by Mary Enig and Sally Fallon.[15] In "The Oiling of America," the authors offer a provocative and illuminating explanation of why the natural fats of our past diet-- the butter, whole milk, lard and tallow--have been almost completely replaced in our society by the unnatural, highly processed vegetable oils, loaded with the trans fats, that are now competing with cholesterol as public health enemy No. 1.

Of particular interest is Enig and Fallon's account of the famous heart surgeon, Dr. Dudley White, and his stance on the diet controversy. The "prudent diet" proponents of the low fat/cholesterol juggernaut crushed his 1956 nationally televised plea for nutritional common sense into oblivion. Dr. White noted that heart disease in the form of myocardial infarction (MI) was non-existent in 1900 when egg consumption was high and corn oil was unavailable. When pressed to support the prudent diet, he replied, "See here, I began my practice as a cardiologist in 1921 and never saw a myocardial infarction patient until 1928. Back in the MI-free days before 1920, the fats were butter and lard, and I think we would all benefit from the kind of diet that we had at a time when no one had ever heard of corn oil." Today most people have forgotten all about Dr. Dudley White and his prophetic words of advice but we are now in a dietary revolution, and the natural fats of our grandparents are rightfully back in vogue in most of the cholesterol restrictive diets reviewed by Kauffman.

However, the Heart Revolution Diet outlined in Dr. McCully's book, *The Heart Revolution*,[16] reflecting, as it does, his vast clinical research and conclusions, prompted me to focus on his dietary recommendations for the purpose of this book.

Dr. McCully's persistent, even tenacious, adherence to his almost "Eureka" concept of homocysteine toxicity causation of arteriosclerosis has gained wide acceptance from researchers in the field. From his first lonely review of arteriosclerotic changes in children who died from genetically pre-ordained homocystinuria, he now seems to have proven his point: cholesterol is not the cause of arteriosclerosis, homocysteine elevation secondary to vitamin deficiency appears to be the major player. Needless to say, to depart so radically from prevailing concepts takes a man with determination but it does not stop there.

McCully's historic work also points to vitamin deficiencies as playing the primary contributory role in arteriosclerosis. Homocysteine, the new villain, becomes predictably elevated in the body only when one or more of the B complex vitamins--folic acid, B6 or B12--are deficient. Arteriosclerosis, it would seem, is a deficiency disease, which, according to McCully (and now many others) makes it potentially treatable by dietary supplementation. Cholesterol is not completely off the hook but its role, when sufficiently elevated, has now become a passive one, that of contributing to the pre-existing arterial disease. Most authorities now accept these findings but are quick to point out homocysteine elevation, by itself, cannot account for all arteriosclerosis and atherosclerosis observed.

As presented by Fallon and Enig in their paper on heart disease causation[17] and Kauffman in his review on supplements,[18] other factors such as trans fats, omega 6, magnesium, oxidants, platelet malfunction, and even low levels of Coenzyme Q10 may be involved.,. Certainly the concept of vitamin or mineral deficiencies as a cause or a significant contributor to public ill health is not new, but this major departure from traditional thinking, thanks in part to Dr. McCully's untiring efforts, now has widespread research support.

A brief review of "nutritional milestones" in the United States and throughout the world reveals a number of instances where a seemingly simple, common and completely ordinary substance has been found to be absolutely vital to our health and well being. Many of these have become part of the basic health curriculum now taught in our schools.

Beriberi, a disease in which degeneration of the nerves leads to heart failure, is caused by a vitamin B1 deficiency. Beriberi reached epidemic proportions in Indonesia and India in the 1900s when rice processing began. Rice in its original form has a husk rich in vitamin B1, and when processing removed this husk, the populations in Indonesia and India suddenly lost their major source of vitamin B1. The solution? White rice must now be fortified with B1.

Scurvy, caused by lack of vitamin C, was a major problem in the fifteenth and sixteenth centuries. With no fresh fruit, vegetables or meat on board, sailors and explorers on long sea voyages were particularly hard hit by the disease.

Pellagra is another vitamin deficiency disease formerly common in our country. In the early 1900s many Southerners subsisted largely on white corn hominy which was devoid of vitamin B3, a vitamin commonly known as niacin. Every freshman medical student quickly learns the three Ds of pellagra: dementia, diarrhea and dermatitis. Now processed corn is fortified with niacin and the disease is practically unheard of.

Iodine's role in goiter prevention and iron's role in the formation of red blood cells have long been common knowledge.

Now, another deficiency state with major repercussions must be added to this impressive list. The big killer, arteriosclerosis--and its offspring, atherosclerosis-- results from subtle deficiencies of such substances as folic acid, B6 and B12, the lack of which leads to toxic elevation of homocysteine levels.

McCully makes his case well, for these common substances--so vital to our ability to metabolize homocysteine--are not only exquisitely sensitive to our techniques of food preparation and processing but often become progressively less available to our bodies as we age. It can be stated unequivocally that despite the abundance of food in our burgeoning supermarkets, we are a nation of individuals largely compromised by subtle deficiencies of folic acid, vitamins B6 and B12. The result is rampant arterial disease with its heart attacks and strokes, our most common cause of death and disability. It seems ironic that a country so favored with such a rich array of resources can suffer diseases caused by something so prosaic as completely preventable vitamin deficiencies. Any doctor worth his salt in public health administration and delivery of health care cringes at the thought.

McCully also reports in *The Heart Revolution* [19] that some 10-40 percent of patients with vascular disease in clinics and hospitals worldwide are shown to have high levels of homocysteine. The well-known Framingham Heart Study has determined that up to two-thirds of the elderly are deficient in B6, B12 or folic acid.

He adds: In February 1998, investigators at the Harvard School of Public Health published the results of the Nurses Health Study. During a fourteen-year period, involving 80,000 participants, those nurses with the lowest consumption of folic acid and B6 had the highest rates of cardiovascular disease and heart attack.

In the 1996 Nutrition Canada Study of 5,000 people studied for fourteen years, those with the lowest levels of folic acid in the blood were almost twice as likely to die from heart disease as were those with the highest levels.

About 12 percent of the population worldwide carries a genetic defect for an enzyme which affects their normal ability to metabolize homocysteine. People born with an abnormality of this enzyme need to consume more folic acid than usual to keep their homocysteine levels in check and thereby reduce the greater associated risk of developing arteriosclerosis and heart disease.

If we now agree that McCully and his growing host of homocysteine researchers have proven their point that elevation of this amino acid is the trigger of the very first abnormal changes in the walls of our arteries--those infamous lipid streaks and foam cells, those glaring signposts of arteriosclerosis to come, noted so commonly in autopsies of young military men killed in action in Korea and Vietnam--we can only ask, "Why haven't the necessary amounts of these magic vitamins been added to our foods for the specific purpose of controlling coronary artery disease?"

When asked if the FDA has done anything about correcting this omission or, at the very least, if they have taken any measures to do so, the answer is an emphatic, "No!" No supplement has been added or is scheduled to be added for the specific purpose of controlling coronary artery disease. Why this is not being done requires a lengthy explanation of the FDA's archaic mechanisms for action on the subject of adding supplements to our processed foodstuffs. McCully reminds us that one does not talk of such progress in years; it is measured in decades.

As we all know, the assurance of the quality of the United States food supply is the primary function of the Food and Drug Administration. In making its decisions, the FDA considers the recommendations of the Food and Nutrition Board of the National Research Council, which is responsible for determining the recommended daily allowances (RDAs) for each nutrient. The FDA also considers the results of current surveys analyzing food consumption, such as the Nationwide Food Consumption Survey, the Continuing Survey of Food Intakes of Individuals, and the National Health and Nutrition Examination Surveys, all sponsored by the U.S. Department of Agriculture. Finally the FDA takes into account the opinions of nationally recognized experts in nutritional science. Predictably, the decision process is so complex that it happens at a glacial pace.

One can imagine McCully's frustration with this sobering reality. To hammer in the point he tells us of the Type Ten Formula proposed to the FDA in 1974 by our National Academy of Sciences and the National Research Council. We already had thiamin, riboflavin, niacin and iron in our cereal as a result of a ponderous FDA mandate of 1941. Then, in 1974, six more supplements were proposed for this list: pyridoxine (B6), folic acid, vitamin A, calcium, magnesium and zinc--a simple enough request, loaded with justification. In 1998 the FDA mandated addition of folic acid to enriched grain foods such as wheat flour and rice. This action was taken to prevent neural tube birth defects. Elevation of homocysteine recently has been associated with human congenital heart disease, club foot, cleft palate and other serious birth defects. The FDA did, at that time, consider the possible additional benefit of homocysteine reduction through folic acid supplementation for the prevention of vascular disease but concluded that the evidence then was insufficient for definitive conclusion. In the year 2002, as of this writing, despite abundant proof that these vital substances are very substantially depleted during food processing, some of them are still awaiting FDA decision and action.

The FDA's inaction on the vitamin supplementation issues was another factor in our recommendation of McCully's Heart Revolution Diet. In his discussion of the carbohydrate restrictive diet, McCully devotes special attention to foods that have abundant amounts of folic acid and the B6 and B12 vitamins so important for holding homocysteine in check. He also advises the necessary cooking techniques that minimize the loss of these substances during food preparation. He generally goes along with the mid-section of the Food Pyramid but recommends a few modifications. Although milk, cheese and yogurt are good sources of calcium and protein and the recommendation to eat two or three servings per day is valid, he takes issue with the recommendation to eat only low fat or fat free products. He is concerned about the associated risk of deficiency of fat-soluble vitamins, since these nutrients are found only in the fat portion of the foods we eat.

Another area McCully would modify is the FDA recommendation to consume two or three servings of meat, poultry, fish, dry beans, eggs or nuts a day. Putting beans and nuts in this group is problematic, he says, because it suggests that plant and animal proteins are interchangeable: "The truth is that plant protein, lacking in the essential amino acids, is quite different from animal protein, which contains plentiful essential amino acids. Therefore, depending only on plants for protein is not a good idea because the protein is inferior." He suggests a daily intake of two or three servings of protein from fish, meats, poultry, eggs or cheese.

He agrees with eating more vegetables and fruits, which are an excellent source of vitamins, minerals, fiber and complex carbohydrates, but reminds us that although "carbohydrates are essential we must choose beneficial carbohydrates-- fruits, vegetables and whole grains--not refined carbohydrates like sugar and flour products." He deplores the tendency of so many Americans to turn to highly refined, vitamin and mineral depleted, readily available, processed foods which, for the most part, tend to be high in refined carbohydrates. As stated earlier, that excessive reliance on such carbohydrates in our diet has lead to the present carbohydrate catastrophe, the obesity epidemic.

McCully's diet is simple: Protein in the form of meat, fish, poultry, eggs, milk, and cheese should comprise about 25 percent of our daily caloric intake. Another 25 to 30 percent should come from the consumption of fats, which includes the fat of ingested meats plus olive oil, butter and cream. The remaining 45-50 percent of our daily caloric intake should be derived from the consumption of complex carbohydrates in the form of fruit, vegetables and whole grains. Balance is key in this diet, primary to maintaining balance in the body.

You won't find Oreos or white bread or french fries in McCully's diet but you will find some remarkable similarities to the food nutritionists who postulate what our diet must have been like 10,000 years ago. Not only has McCully focused his diet on the prevention of arteriosclerosis but he also presents a diet to which we are already well suited, genetically speaking. We are still hunter-gathers like our forebears, he says, but we must now confine our searches to the aisles of supermarkets in our quest for just the right foods.

Not only does McCully's diet help keep homocysteine levels comfortably in the normal range, lessening the possibility of damage to the lining of our arteries, it also seems to be just as effective as the low cholesterol/low fat diet for normalizing serum cholesterol, a subject of immense concern to today's patients, despite the lack of any significant association with cardiovascular disease. If one's arteries are not primed with lipid streaks and foam cells, LDL remains in its largely unoxidized form, and cholesterol deposition into incipient atheroma becomes unlikely.

Hopefully, I have answered the question readers might have asked earlier, "Why all this focus on diet and cholesterol when this book started out to be about amnesia and memory dysfunction associated with statin drug use?" It is a logical progression if significant findings necessary for improved patient health are to be understood and put into practice.

The overwhelming majority of people in our country today have been taught to regard cholesterol as the villain in coronary heart disease. Understandably, they have been led to consider the American Heart Association's low cholesterol/ low fat diet as the correct choice for keeping cholesterol levels in check. Because of this, they have become fair game for the promoters of broader and broader utilization of the statin class of drugs to reduce cholesterol levels. The reality that almost all major intervention studies have failed to find a significant correlation of serum cholesterol levels with cardiovascular diseases has fallen on ears deafened by drug promotional literature. Most individuals with the risk factors of hypertension, obesity, smoking and positive family history for arteriosclerosis now consider themselves to be suitable candidates for statin drug intervention despite their frequently modest cholesterol and LDL levels. This makes the job of those promoting wider use of statin drugs even easier.

But I have learned that cholesterol is not the villain in arteriosclerosis--other factors are, primary of which is homocysteine--and our extraordinary efforts over the past fifty years to adhere to a low fat/ low cholesterol diet appear to have been misdirected. This recent evidence suggests, even demands, a radical departure from our dependency on a misguided "national" diet that not only has failed to nourish and protect our health but also has actively undermined it. We need a new diet that is far more restrictive with respect to the consumption of simple carbohydrates and processed foodstuffs that have been stripped of vitally important vitamins and minerals. Authorities are surely beginning to realize that, had we taken this path fifty years ago, our current dependence on statin drugs for control of heart disease and stroke would be substantially reduced, if not eliminated.

It is for this reason that I felt compelled to include social emphasis on diet in our presentation of transient global amnesia and other forms of memory dysfunction associated with statin drug use. McCully has given us reason to believe that, while cholesterol is an absolutely vital substance, it is innocuous in its natural, unoxidized form. Its passive involvement as a component in sclerotic plaques occurs only because of pre-existing factors completely unrelated to cholesterol. If we are to rationally approach the problems of prevention of arteriosclerosis and its secondary complications of heart disease and stroke and excessive dependence on statin drugs, we need to recognize the full array of nutritional factors that are contributing. To accomplish this, medication and proper diet must go hand in hand. Together, they can become a very effective "double whammy" in the prevention and treatment of arteriosclerosis and its complications.

Applying these concepts one can look toward a future with a greatly reduced need for statin drug use. Our memories are far too precious to risk compromise. Do we really have a choice?

Transient global amnesia is probably as old as man and, as we have suggested, statin drugs may be just the latest of its many triggers. However, its varied reactions--vague preservation of identity, maddeningly repetitive questioning, absolute inability to preserve new memories and, in some cases, retrograde memory lapses decades into the past--can be subtle and elusive. But, as so poignantly described in Chapter I and in the following case report, regardless of which trigger provokes an attack--cold water, emotional stress, exercise, sex, cerebral angiography or statin drugs-- the psychological impact on the patient is devastating.

"I was on four different statins for a period of over 10 years, on dosages from 10 mg to 80 mg. I had muscle pain and cramps for a number of years, and I put it down to aging or muscle strain. This was while I was on 10 mg to 40 mg. In July of 2002 I was on 40 mg of Pravachol, and after blood tests showed [my] cholesterol was over 400, I was placed on 80 mg of Lipitor. And that is when the nightmare began. Although the pain from muscle spasms and cramps had become so bad that I took early retirement in 2001 because I could not get through the day, I had never had problems with memory or cognitive functions before. I did not suspect statin drug toxicity until April 2003 when my husband suggested to my neurologist that I come off all meds

for two weeks to see if that would help. At that time the only way I could walk was with a cane or a walker to keep myself from falling. I had very little muscle tone in the calves of my legs, and my legs would just suddenly give way under me. And the pain was terrible.

Since going on the Lipitor in July 2002, I have had four episodes of disoriented thinking, confusion and lost time. The last time occurred 6 August 2003 and lasted approximately 2 to 3 hours. The time before, I lost about 5 hours and that occurred on 22 June 2003.My husband and daughter took me to the ER that time.

I am so tired of defending myself from doctors who feel my problems do not have anything to do with the statins, and that everything that happened to me is "mental". I am at the point of not going back to see my primary care physician again or any other specialist. I definitely will not take their statins!"

This patient has been devastated--emotionally, physically and mentally--by her experiences with statin drug use over the past 10 years. Clearly, she has experienced disabling physical symptoms but, in addition, she reports 4 amnesia episodes. She is an excellent example of the medical community's failure to recognize the full spectrum of statin drug side effects and to understand that many of them are irreversible.

Statin drugs, as they currently exist, interfere with cholesterol biosynthesis at the HMG-CoA reductase step and, as a consequence, inevitably must interfere with ubiquinone and dolichol production, processes vital for cell integrity and maintenance. This can only be called collateral damage, a very serious consideration, since most of the side effects we are seeing are secondary to this collateral damage. On the other hand, the absolute requirement for cholesterol's biosynthesis by the glial cells for synapse formation and function suggests a strong possibility that statin drugs might interfere directly at the brain cell, as well as at the better understood hepatic cell level. Cognitive problems seem almost inevitable with interference at the glial cell level.

It is impossible to hide my frustration that now, long after patient case reports first began to surface, the average practicing physician in this country is still completely unaware that serious cognitive side effects can be associated with statin drug use. Many of those reports tell of doctors who all too often jump immediately to the presumptive diagnosis of "senior moments," approaching senility or possibly even early Alzheimer's, when apprised of memory gaps and increasing confusion in the patient. Frequently, the last thing considered, if, indeed, the doctor thinks of it at all, is a reaction to the patient's statin drug. One of my aims in writing this book and heightening the awareness of both doctors and patients will be realized when doctors first consider statin side effects as the genesis of their bewildered patient's symptoms and then reduce the dosage or seek an alternative therapy.

Doctors must also remember that such side effects do not necessarily become apparent only in the first few months of statin therapy. Some of the most serious side effects reported have presented after an interval of three or four trouble-free years of statin use, so constant vigilance is necessary. Patients all too frequently accept erosion of memory and increasing tendency for confusion and disorientation as an inevitable consequence of aging. They, too, often need to be reminded that not all memory problems are age related and that they as well as their doctors must always consider a medication's side effects when cognitive problems appear.

And there *are* two sides to the cholesterol issue. This notorious, Janus-faced substance is both a component of atherosclerotic plaque and, at the same time, one of the most important substances in our body. In its first guise, there is no doubt that cholesterol is found in atheroma but it is not the cause of the underlying arterial disease. McCulley[1] helped pave the way--and other researchers are following--when he determined that homocysteine, by allowing lipid/mucoid 'streaks' and inflammatory cells to accumulate in those fragile tissues lining the arteries, is the initial trigger of arteriosclerosis. Cholesterol is a more or less passive bystander, streaming by these damaged areas within its lipoprotein carrier and occasionally deposited by errant LDL, misguided in its alien, "oxidized" form. Gobbled up by a wandering phagocyte, the complex becomes the ominous "foam cell" and the process of hardening of the arteries with plaque formation is underway. *With or without excess cholesterol the process of arteriosclerosis can and does take place in arteries.*

When doctors use statin drugs for control of cholesterol values, they must be made aware that the unpleasant, serious and even lethal side effect profile of these drugs includes the previously unrecognized symptom complex of transient global amnesia and extreme forgetfulness, disorientation and confusion. These cognitive effects mirror an inability to remember who we are and, unfortunately, are not identified as the drug side effects they are. It is very important that physicians make their patients aware of these possible reactions. Most practicing physicians are well aware of the statin drugs' tendency to cause liver toxicity, polyneuropathy and rhabdomyolysis, but impairment of memory is so novel that these drugs are being prescribed for the pilots and other aircrew members of our high performance fighter jets and passenger transport aircraft. The physicians making these decisions have never been apprised of the possibility that a pilot may, with no warning, suddenly regress to his teen-age years, the period long before he learned to fly.

The other face of cholesterol in the human body is the vital one and well deserving of the emphasis we have given it. The astounding importance of this ubiquitous substance in cellular membrane function and in synaptic formation and function, so recently discovered by Pfrieger[2] and his colleagues, serves to illustrate just how critical cholesterol is at the cellular level.

Strong statins such as Lipitor, Mevacor and Zocor have the capacity to cause major reductions in serum cholesterol values. Many patients proudly announce that their cholesterol plummeted "from 280 to 160" in a matter of weeks, attesting to the spectacular effectiveness of these stronger statins in some patients, but we must remember that the statins tend to be lipophilic, easily traversing the so-called blood brain barrier, which for these statins is no barrier at all. Dr. Beatrice Golomb, of UCSD's Department of Medicine, reports that in her case studies of transient global amnesia patients,[3] cholesterol reductions of this magnitude were very common. Such evidence suggests that abrupt, major decreases of serum cholesterol from statin drug therapy should be taken more as a warning than as an indication of success, for cognitive side effects seemed more likely to occur in these cases. When the practicing physician, who, despite the paucity of supportive research data, has determined that the use of statin drugs for cholesterol control is justified, is faced with this type of response, consideration should be given to prompt reduction in statin drug dosage of these patients, followed by more gradual titration to the lowest possible effective dose. Such patients are unusually sensitive to the statin class of drugs and special attention to dosage is required to minimize side effects. For many medications, one-half or one-quarter of the recommended starting dose may be completely adequate for patients, Dr.

Jay Cohen[4] advises, and this lower amount will give comparable results with fewer side effects. The statin drugs, if used for cholesterol control, are no exception and the dosages are cumulative in their effect. The longer even the smaller doses are taken by a patient, however, the more potent they can become, and care must be exercised on an on-going basis to further reduce even maintenance doses if necessary. With all drugs, doctors should prescribe the smallest dose possible that will achieve the desirable goal of reasonable control.

Defining reasonable control of serum cholesterol levels is not easy in light of the failure of study after study to show a significant effect on all cause mortality. An excellent review of this dilemma is presented by John Allred in his review article on lowering serum cholesterol.[5] In light of our present knowledge of cholesterol's largely passive role in arteriosclerosis and the very substantial side effect risks from the stronger statin drugs, attempts to reduce the risk of cardiovascular disease by cholesterol control may be counterproductive for many patients. This may be particularly true in patients who have no other serious medical issues.

I naturally focused my attention on diet, as the shift in scientific thinking toward homocysteine elevation as the cause of arteriosclerosis, and the importance of folic acid, B6 and B12 in controlling homocysteine levels in the body became evident. The "national" low cholesterol/low fat diet has failed not only its original intent to control arteriosclerosis and its consequences, it has actually fueled Type 2 diabetes and obesity epidemics in this country. In its race to produce low cholesterol and low fat products to satisfy the national diet, the food industry has delivered a superabundance of refined carbohydrates and nutrient-depleted foodstuffs that have exacerbated the problem. Instead of healthier, we have become a generation of pathetically "fattened sheep," prey to diabetes, stroke, heart attack, and worsening arteriosclerosis.

For these very real dietary reasons, I have stressed the importance of Dr. Kilmer McCully's research efforts over the past decades and his vision, shared by many others, that a very substantial reduction in the prevalence and severity of arteriosclerosis is possible from dietary supplementation alone. Large-scale studies currently underway suggest they are correct. I feel a future of implementing a diet based the findings of these scientists will substantially lower cardiovascular disease and the need for medication. Diet and proper nutrition also holds the promise for reversing the rising tide of Type 2 diabetes in adults, a tide that is now also afflicting young children. The problem is becoming so acute in the West and in some Asian developing countries that doctors consider being grossly overweight and the high risk of contracting diabetes to be intimately connected. So much so that a new term "diabesity," a blend of "diabetes" and "obesity," has been coined to sum up the escalating problem.

Elevated cholesterol is not the problem we have been led to believe. Yes it is a component of atherosclerotic plaque but a passive one. As McCully has stated, our present emphasis on cholesterol control requires dispassionate reassessment. Based on the myriad problems associated with low cholesterol levels that we have reported, some would state that low cholesterol is more of a problem than high cholesterol. A decade ago such a statement would have clearly been a joke, but today the research evidence gives compelling support to its truth..

Just as McCully's work has been very influential in my research for this book, so can it be a vital resource for the many health organizations in our country that are involved in making dietary decisions. We need new dietary guidelines for the public and the food industry. We need to get back to basics in the field of nutrition. There is reason to believe that a national diet more liberal in protein and certain natural fats and far more restrictive in refined (or any) carbohydrates would be a major step forward. A number of excellent dietary guidelines of this type are available but Dr. McCully's Heart Revolution Diet[6] is given special consideration in this book because of its focus on homocysteine and nutritional deficiencies as the etiologic agents in arteriosclerosis.

And, finally, now knowing cholesterol's critical role in brain function and being aware of the dangers that can result when that process is interrupted or circumvented, I am incredulous that statin drugs are proposed so liberally. So much of what we are completely dependent upon is reliant on the so-called HMG-COA reductase process--the point of attack of the statin drugs and the target of the pharmaceutical industry in their zeal for cholesterol control--that our memories, our sexuality, our metabolism, our very life is threatened by disruption of the process at this point.

The present trend toward broader and broader use of statin drugs must be re-evaluated in light of the very compelling evidence that lowering cholesterol is not the solution to lowering the devastating effects of arteriosclerosis. There is no better time than now to challenge this national usage trend. The statin drugs are not without risk. Certainly the many deaths from rhabdomyolysis clearly point to serious and unpredictable risk. And these deaths are still occurring, despite the FDA's belated recall of Baycol®. The cognitive side effects such as amnesia and memory loss are of particular interest, not only because of the many cases already reported but also for those cases that will never be reported because they are too subtle. They are lost forever in that wasteland of forgotten things in the mind, mistakenly presumed to be part of our heritage of imprecision and the best our memories can do. In other words, it is likely that the reported cognitive events are but the tip of the iceberg in regard to the true incidence of statin "costs." Our memory is so important to us that any hint of threat, particularly from drugs that were prescribed for a totally unrelated medical condition, strikes at the very core of our being.

"What other recourse do we have?" ask the cardiologists and the primary care physicians, beleaguered by the pharmaceutical industry, the dictates of organized medicine, peer pressure and patient demands and fueled by direct-to-patient advertising. "Statins are all we have."

Lee of the Thrombosis and Vascular Biology Unit of Birmingham's City Hospital in the UK, would say omega 3 and he brilliantly presents his documentation;[7] Coenzyme Q10 say the Langsjoens in their overview of the use of Coenzyme Q10 in cardiovascular disease.[8] The benefits of vitamin E and magnesium are referenced by Kauffman in his review of aspiring compared with other modalities for both primary and secondary prevention of cardiovascular disease.[9] Lower homocysteine would be the advice of Kilmer McCully, stressing the prevalence of subtle deficiencies of vitamins B6 and B12 and folic acid in our over-nourished society.

The drug companies say, "Use our statins," with decreasing regard for cholesterol levels and increasing emphasis on the newly recognized anti-inflammatory action of these drugs. If statins are a super-aspirin it must be so stated. Promotional literature must turn away from current emphasis on cholesterol control for that does not appear to be our problem, arteriosclerosis control is, and inflammation of arterial linings is a well documented factor in plaque formation. A super-aspirin is needed but one with an acceptable side effect profile. The side effects of current statin drugs seriously limit justification for use for primary prevention. Much more developmental work is necessary to perfect a suitable class of drugs for this purpose.

Studies that explore the use of statin drugs for stroke and heart attack prevention have yielded extraordinarily inconsistent findings. The truly comprehensive study conducted by Dr. Collins[10] of Oxford University proved that his heart patients lowered their risk of heart attacks and strokes by one-third after taking statins. On the basis of such seemingly positive findings, Dr. Collins estimates that an additional 200 million persons worldwide could benefit from this drug that he considers the "new aspirin" for warding off heart trouble.

Yet, Dr. Joel M. Kauffman, reporting on a long-term study by Jackson, et al,[11] finds that long-term use of statins for primary prevention of heart disease produced a 1 percent greater risk of death over 10 years vs. placebo, when the results of all the big controlled trials reported before 2000 were combined. Dr. Kauffman noted further that even for short-term use, 16 weeks in the MIRACL study by Schwartz, et al,[12] in patients with heart or angina problems, the use of Lipitor (atorvastatin) at a rich 80 mg/day did not significantly change the all cause death rate or the rate of heart attacks. Such inconsistencies naturally make interpretation of these kinds of data extremely difficult and underscores the crucial need for the members of the pharmaceutical industry to make patient safety their primary priority, since side effects are probable and benefit is not.

That the cognitive side effect problems of the statin drugs are just being recognized in the utilization of these drugs is a direct result of the current flawed research and dysinformation processes of the pharmaceutical companies. The incomplete and misleading information currently being distributed to doctors and patients as a result of those flawed processes has created a vacuum of awareness of the potential memory problems even as it almost guarantees an enormous profit return. In fact, in 2003, Pfizer's Lipitor is expected to become the first $10 billion drug in history.[13]

The FDA must initiate, with congressional support, a complete revamping and revitalization of its policies for approval and distribution of the pharmaceutical industries' drugs and products. This initiative must define patient safety as the primary reason for the FDA's very existence. It must also resist any and all industry efforts to fast track their medications for approval in order to insure that company's market share. It should request and welcome the establishment of an independent National Medications Safety Board, funded by the pharmaceutical industry, to oversee the safety of post-approval medications and all other aspects of the drug industry.

Even more importantly, the pharmaceutical industry must be compelled to conform to the same high ethics in the production and marketing of their products that physicians are held to. They need to be made aware of the consequences of their pursuit for exorbitant market and profit return at the cost of mounting loss of patient and doctor confidence. The extraordinarily high pedestal most patients place their doctors on deserves that equally high standards are defined and maintained for the medications those doctors dispense. The annual toll of lives and serious side effects currently sustained by hundreds of thousands of patients is a heavy and unnecessary price to pay for faith misplaced.

And looming large in the near future is the very real possibility of "pay back" time for the pharmaceutical companies. The current class action law suits being tried in American courts as a result of the statin drug, Baycol, and its lethal side effects in the death of dozens of patients appears to be just the beginning. Those hidden side effects of Baycol before the FDA finally recalled it are being noted by some of the nation's top plaintiff's attorneys as they train their sites on the drug industry. After successfully fighting the asbestos and tobacco companies, these attorneys are ready to claim that many giant pharmaceutical companies, in hiding the dangers of their medicines, have harmed thousands of people.

An indisputable, ironic double loss occurs when half of the patients in this country discontinue urgently needed medications because of preventable side effects. "The patient loses by becoming exposed to markedly increased risks of premature disease and death," advises Dr. Jay Cohen,[14] and the drug industry loses increased drug sales when patients become dissatisfied with a medication and discontinue treatment.

The attending physician, the patient and the drug industry all lose when drug side effects are unacceptable. This irony is particularly true when these side effects include the theft of our most precious commodity, our very memory.

The End

ADDENDUM:

This Addendum, dealing with the neurophysiologic
mechanisms and differential diagnosis of transient global
amnesia, was prepared specifically for practicing physicians to
aid in their management of this often obscure condition. The lay
reader may find much of this information difficult to assimilate.
However, included are selected case histories of value to both lay
and professional readers. .I recommend that the lay reader at least
scan this material.

Part I
<u>Mechanisms of Transient Global Amnesia</u>

Transient global amnesia is not new, nor is it a medical
malady that has 'arrived' recently due to increasingly sophisticated
medical diagnostic ability. For nearly fifty years researchers have
been attempting to discover the underlying cause. Today, despite
the availability of imaging technology not even dreamed of five
decades ago, lack of agreement still exists as to the precise factors
involved. Each of the several possible mechanisms has had its
share of ardent and strong-willed advocates. Many firmly believe
that the vasospastic etiology of migraine explains it all, by
pointing to the large numbers of cases where various imaging
techniques have revealed indisputable evidence of diminished
blood flow in those areas of the brain known to be involved in
memory processing and retrieval. Others, at one time or another,
have pointed to epilepsy as the trigger mechanism, offering
various explanations as to why the EEGs in classic global amnesia
cases are consistently free of epileptiform activity. Admittedly, the
well-known amnesic aura of epilepsy comes extraordinarily close
in clinical presentation to classic transient global amnesia. Still
others point to cerebrovascular factors comparable to those
causing transient ischemic attacks as responsible. If so, the cause
might be a loose cluster of platelets cells clinging together
sufficiently long to transiently block circulation before breaking
up and reverting to normal blood flow. Closely related to this is
the possibility that venous congestion may be contributory. Lewis[1]
has proposed that venous congestion, by causing disruption of
blood flow to key brain structures, may help explain the unusual

148

association of strenuous exercise, highly active sex, cold water immersion, and the Valsalva maneuver with transient global amnesia attacks. For similar reasons others have suggested that whatever elevates intrathoracic pressure inevitably contributes to venous congestion with its possible sequellae.

This would appear to be the logical place to discuss another possible contributor to this tempest of interrelating physical and biological factors: patent foramen ovale. Most readers have never heard of this vital structure that is the source of our ability to live while completely immersed in liquid. Throughout the nine months we float about in the amniotic fluid of our mother's uterus, breathing in the normal sense is impossible. Our lungs have no function in this environment. Mother Nature benevolently decreed we should bypass the lungs during our "underwater"gestation.

Venous blood entering the right atrium of the heart is diverted from the lungs directly into the comparable chamber on the left side of the heart, through our patent foramen ovale. This subject of circulation of blood in the fetus is a fascinating one but, other than for the foramen ovale, not relevant to the subject of transient global amnesia. What is relevant, however, is the astonishing frequency wherein this life-giving opening fails to close securely after our first few breaths, when it no longer is needed. This subject has intrigued researchers in the field of cerebrovascular accidents and Homma[2] reports that approximately 40 per cent of cerebral infarctions that cannot be classified as strokes of determined cause, despite a complete diagnostic work-up, are labeled as "cryptogenic strokes." Contrast echocardiography in such patients has revealed an extremely high incidence of patent foramen ovale, with values as high as 40 percent. Of particular interest are the values ranging from 20 to 55 percent for transient global amnesia patients. Precise data on the incidence of this finding in the general public are difficult to obtain but it has been estimated to be as high as 10 percent.

The incidence of this abnormality has come to light only in the past several decades, as imaging technology has become both more precise and available. But the impact is a sobering awareness that many of us have patent foramen ovale and, with it, the potential for the same right to left shunting of blood that made our fetal lives possible. The problem is that as adults we carry the risk that emboli of one type of another can now pass directly into our brains. We have lost the "safety net" of having our venous blood thoroughly filtered by our lungs.

So far, none of this would seem to have any bearing on the effect of statin drugs on memory and other cognitive functions, but since there are two sides to every coin, there is an opposite side to this right-to-left shunt that is very relevant. To have this right to left shunt presupposes that on occasion the pressure within the right atrial chamber exceeds that of the left. When this point is reached, venous blood, platelet emboli, nitrogen bubbles or "what have you" pass over to their destiny on the left side of the body. Anything that raises venous pressure, be it vigorous sex, strenuous exercise, performing the Valsalva maneuver for your doctor, positive pressure breathing with a mask as in diving and high altitude vacuum chambers, or in vigorous coughing--the possibilities are many--produces the same results. But what of the other times, when you are resting? This is when you have the left to right shunt because the pressure on the left ordinarily greatly exceeds the right. The shunt of blood may not be much, perhaps just a few cubic centimeters every heartbeat, but it is still easily enough to raise venous pressure above normal and keep it there. The result is venous congestion, creating potential interference with blood flow and tissue metabolism upstream, which is analogous to building a dam across a stream with predictable consequences to the flow of water. Lewis's interesting concept of venous pressure as a trigger to transient global amnesia becomes much more interesting when one considers the reality that many of us may have patent foramen ovale.

Since we are on the subject of plumbing variations and their not so subtle effects on circulation, what of the well-known subclavian steal syndrome? Using the old adage of "robbing Peter to pay Paul," we can simplify the explanation. With society's awareness of the DNA mandated differences that make each of us so unique, it is not surprising to learn of the many different ways arterial blood is carried to our heads and brain. In many of us the right vertebral artery branches from our subclavian artery rather than directly from the aorta. As some of you know, our subclavian artery supplies our arm (Paul) and our vertebral artery connects with other arteries in the brain (Peter). The "steal" part occurs when vigorous arm activity demands more blood than the subclavian can supply from its origin at the aorta. It then "steals" from the vertebral, depriving the brain of sufficient blood and

150

oxygen during the arm exercise. This becomes particularly interesting when one learns that the stolen blood was originally intended to supply brain tissue involved in memory. Whether from diminished arterial flow or congestion of venous return from increased pressure, the ischemic results on the tissues involved can be quite comparable.

Only one other possibility of any merit remains--spreading depression, a condition that is described by some as the electrochemical equivalent of surgical ablation. Once triggered, this deactivation process slowly sweeps across the involved area of brain tissue causing oxygen and glucose uptake to all but cease while creating a sharp rise of extracellular potassium and precipitous falls of both sodium and chloride. From the viewpoint of a cell this is serious business, indeed, for the energy of a cell is completely dependent upon the balance of these ions. Potassium ions on the outside of a cell wall are like an uncharged battery. We are dealing with a slowly spreading area of tissue depleted of the very stuff of life. Then, into this all but dead zone of brain tissue flows a massive influx of calcium and the condition rapidly can become a life or death matter. Fortunately, recovery is the rule where the trigger agent is transient, and the body slowly reverses the process. Those studying animal models of stroke can control whether or not tissue death will occur simply by juggling the acidity levels and the balance of these ions.

Fortunately, in our classic transient global amnesia cases, Mother Nature remains firmly in control. A vasospastic insult or a fleeting thromboembolic one may trigger spreading depression, preventing for a time the laying down of new memories or recovery of past ones, but it remains transitory, resolving within twenty-four hours. This proposed mechanism for transient global amnesia is rapidly gaining acceptance as research data present an ever more convincing case. Interestingly, this process closely resembles the much more serious sequence of events seen in stroke, either ischemic or hemorrhagic. The end result is ischemia of brain tissue, triggering spreading depression. Whether recovery or death ensues depends entirely on the degree and duration of ischemia.

Migraine is a class of recurrent headaches so common that nearly everyone has heard of them. Occasionally the headache is preceded by an "aura." The aura typically involves visual changes, such as seeing wavy lines, spots or even hallucinations. Auras

151

have been consistently tied to a phenomenon known as cortical spreading depression, during which a wave of altered brain activity sweeps across the cortex of the brain. Frank Richter,[3] reported on the failure of cortical spreading depression to fully explain migraine headache, despite offering a firm neurophysiological basis for aura. This would seem to be a process similar, if not identical to, the spreading depression process just described, with the difference being primarily one of location in the brain. If located in the memory structures of the brain, transient global amnesia may result; if the occipital cortex is involved, the auras of migraine follow.

Yes, transient global amnesia is related to migraines and there seems to be some crossing over of neurophysiology but they are different. Only a relatively small percentage of transient global amnesia patients have a migraine history and the triggers, especially the venous pressure feature, are noticeably lacking in migraine.

Returning to the transient global amnesia syndrome and the similarity of signs and symptoms that herald the likely diagnosis to the experienced examiner: why are patients so much alike despite the disparity in age, gender and precipitating factors? The answer would seem to be the final common pathway concept mentioned earlier. The diverse nature of precipitating factors seems to condense to very small numbers when the venous congestion concept is considered. Ischemia of certain of the tissues involved in memory could be the final insult that initiates the potentially harmful spreading depression. It is relevant to consider how the statins fit this paradigm.

Since, as Pfrieger[4] has proven, biosynthesis of cholesterol at the glial cell is imperative for neuronal function and synapse formation, the statin drugs, the HMG-CoA reductase inhibitors, sensitize us, in a manner of speaking, to the slightest hint of altered brain metabolism. Transient spreading depression, tolerable to many as nothing or a minor nuisance, might well be magnified in those in whom neuronal tissue is under the effect of statins. As one hovers on the edge of synaptic competence due to statin drug effect, the slightest hint of impairment of neuronal glucose, or oxygen consumption, or altered ionic balance such as might ensue with spreading depression, might be just sufficient to tilt a patient toward transient global amnesia.

At the time of this writing, spreading depression remains the "best fit" mechanism to explain the "final neurophysiologic pathway" of transient global amnesia. It offers a framework within which one can explain either the milder cases wherein the presenting deficit is primarily anterograde amnesia, or the much more complex cases where both anterograde and retrograde amnesia to the patient's distant past occur. It also offers an explanation for the permanent obliteration of memory occasionally seen, and even for those cases in which several days may be required for recovery. As to trigger factors, venous congestion has definite physiological appeal and certainly fits the observed data quite well. When one considers the added predisposition of those among us with hidden patent foramen ovale or susceptibility to subclavian steal, venous congestion becomes particularly congruous.

Obviously, not all factors hang so comfortably on the venous congestion/ spreading depression framework. What of the "traveler's amnesia" associated with benzodiazapine use? Can this be considered the same as transient global amnesia? Most regard its lack of repetitive questioning and exclusively anterograde qualities as evidence that it is not. The majority considers the altered memory, occasional depersonalization, confusion, and hallucinations as evidence of a central nervous system depressant activity. We must leave the final determination on this to future research.

As mentioned in Chapter II, the quite common association of transient global amnesia with cerebral angiography deserves another question mark as to mechanism. Are tiny emboli released into the carotid artery, secondary to the process of catheter insertion or is the generally alien nature of the solution--definitely not your normal tissue perfusing solution- triggering a sort of mechanical embolization and transiently altering tissue metabolism; or is it a toxic reaction in certain individuals? Any of these choices might conceivably serve to trigger a spreading reaction but at this point must remain conjecture.

Part 2
Differential Diagnosis of Transient Global Amnesia

Although the presence of transient global amnesia is becoming more readily apparent to the experienced diagnostician, a number of other diagnostic possibilities must be considered. They include head injury, epilepsy, brain tumor, CVA, migraine, Wernicke-Korsakoff syndrome, meningitis and encephalitis, hypoglycemia, medications such as benzodiazepines, drugs of abuse, and psychogenic fugue state.

That head trauma can cause a syndrome of symptoms closely resembling transient global amnesia is well documented.[1-3] In most cases, the evidence of head trauma is all too clear. This is perhaps most powerfully exemplified in Schacter's book, *Searching for Memory,*[4] in which he masterfully portrays Gene, who was thirty years old at the time an accident severely damaged large segments of his frontal and temporal lobes, including the left hippocampus. Since that time Gene not only has been unable to formulate any new memories but he cannot remember a single specific episode from any time in his life. Schacter states that asking Gene about his personal past is an almost unnerving experience. Even when primed by detailed descriptions of dramatic events in his life, Gene has not the barest hint of recall and simply does his best to respond politely in his characteristic quiet, affable manner. Schacter describes a life without any episodic memory as psychologically barren, the equivalent of living in a bleak Siberian landscape. Thankfully, the memory impairment of classic global amnesia is mercifully brief, measured in hours rather than the frequently permanent loss resulting from the more severe head injuries.

Of particular interest to my discussion of transient global amnesia, however, is the fact that even relatively mild trauma without loss of consciousness can result in an amnesia state indistinguishable from the classic transient global one. A history of head trauma may be completely lacking in these cases. Without a reliable observer, a patient would have no recall for the fall or blow. In the absence of visible evidence, the reality of trauma might easily be missed. Special vigilance on the part of emergency room doctors is necessary for, in the absence of visible signs of injury and lack of reliable history, head trauma might never be suspected.

154

Epilepsy may take a number of diverse forms. Of special interest here is the so-called amnestic seizure syndrome, nearly indistinguishable from transient global amnesia.[5-12] The similarity has prompted more than one researcher to consider transient global amnesia to have an epileptic basis. This possibility has been extremely difficult to disprove in the presence of normal EEGs and indeterminate response to anti-epileptic drugs. Hodges and Warlock's report of a 7 percent incidence of epilepsy in the first follow-up year of their "classic" transient global amnesia cases further fuels the fire of controversy. In such cases the features that most accurately correlate with the ultimate development of epilepsy are a relatively brief duration, such as 15 minutes or less, and multiplicity of amnesia attacks. When both of these findings are present their combined predictive value is close to 90 percent within the first year of onset. However, despite the eerie and unsettling resemblance of the amnestic epileptic state to transient global amnesia, the consensus seems to be in favor of a non-epileptic origin to this disorder.

Total global amnesia syndrome has been reported as a presenting complaint in a number of cases where subsequent imaging studies have revealed the presence of one or more space occupying lesions.[13-21] In most of these cases, proximity of the growing mass to some component of the brain's memory apparatus has been the triggering factor. Most of the time the mysterious hippocampal areas, the thalamus with its intricate connections throughout the brain and those adjacent, inner portions of the temporal lobes that encase them are the primary areas involved. The transient global amnesia in these cases frequently persists beyond the time criteria usually accepted for "benign" cases and, predictably, multiple attacks occur. Though an uncommon cause of transient global amnesia. the possibility of an underlying space-occupying lesion probably justifies routine imaging in all cases. The underlying nature of the mass is of little import and runs the gamut from vascular malformation and abscess to primary malignancy and metastastic tumor. What is important is a location touching on the well-known pathways and structures involved in memory processing and storage.

Reports of cerebrovascular accidents presenting as transient global amnesia are legion. Bogousslavsky[22] reports four patients with cerebral hemorrhage or an infarct of the medial part of the temporal lobe or thalamus. Goldenberg[23] reported infarction of the thalamus in a 40-year-old man with transient global amnesia of two days duration. Gorelick[24] described thalamic infarction in a patient who later developed persistent amnesia. Greer[25] presented the case of a 77-year-old woman with classic transient global amnesia due to a temporal lobe stroke. Jacome[26] reported a case of frontal lobe hemorrhage affecting hippocampal pathways. Takahashi[27] reported an unusual case of dural arteriovenous fistula, which apparently contributed to congestion of temporal lobes resulting in its presentation as amnesia. Clearly the medial part of the temporal lobes, the thalamus and hippocampus, must be intact and functioning for proper memory retrieval to take place. Naturally, the amnesia syndrome in such cases by definition usually does not meet the accepted criteria for classic transient global amnesia but it is somewhat unsettling in that this ordinarily benign condition can be simulated so closely by life threatening cerebrovascular disease. The following case history is an excellent illustration of the tendency wherein the symptoms of statin associated transient global amnesia are confused with stroke and other brain pathology. The possibility of drug side effect is rarely considered in such cases.

"Last January, while I was working out at the local fitness center, I became disoriented and confused but I was able to drive myself home without any problem. When I arrived home, I called my wife and told her I thought I was having a stroke. She immediately called our next-door neighbor who came over to sit with me until she arrived home. (I'm telling you all of these facts only from what I have been told because I can't remember any of the events that occurred.)

"When my wife arrived home she decided to take me to the emergency room. While turning the car around in the driveway, I asked her why there were certain lines drawn on the asphalt. I didn't remember that I was having the driveway repaired. Then she asked me if I remembered who I was doing consulting work for at the time. I didn't. Even though I had been doing work for them for about two years. (By the way, I'm an aerodynamicist with specialty in gas turbines.) This scared her. So she called an ambulance. The first memory I have after the event was in the emergency room. For the next several hours, time seemed to pass in jerks. I would be talking to my wife or others and look at the clock and 2 or 3 hours would have passed in an apparent instant.

"My wife tells me that during all of this time I carried on normal conversations. So normal, that she and my neighbor thought I might be just playing a joke on them. My wife says that I appeared to be very agitated and kept asking the same questions over and over again. Not remembering the answers I had gotten before.

"I have heart disease and had bypass surgery done in June 1999. Since that time I have been on statin drugs. First it was Baycol until it was withdrawn and then I tried Lipitor, which I couldn't tolerate. Finally, I arrived at Zocor. My cholesterol has never been very high--about 200. My genetic problem seems to be associated with a low HDL. I have seen studies recently that indicated that by combining Zocor with niacin, you could significantly improve your future health. So I, with doctor's consent, added niacin to my medication. This is when I had my event. The confusing part of this comes from the diagnostic tests that were run. A CT scan that was taken shortly after arriving at the hospital showed that I had a small area of the brain that had died. The report from the neurologist indicated that he thought this was an old (congenital?) sign. Since I never had a CT scan before, there was no way of verifying this conclusion. Later I had a MRI. The physician who read this said that he thought the same area was new because the boundaries appeared to be sharp. His conclusion was that I had a stroke caused by an embolism.

"This last week, I had another event. Not as severe this time. I didn't have any memory loss but had the same confusion that I must have initially experienced the first time. Like the last time, I ended up the emergency room. They again did a CT scan and it again showed the small defect. When I asked them about the results from the CT scan and MRI the previous January, they both (independently) said that a CT scan would not show evidence of a stoke when taken within a few hours of the onset of the event. I suppose this might not be the case if the stroke was caused by a hemorrhage. This event is coincident with my increase in the amount of Zocor and niacin the previous month. As you can see, I am now confused about my health status and the medications I am taking. I now believe that these events are associated with the Zocor and niacin rather than a stroke."

This case demonstrates the challenging diagnostic dilemma posed by pre-existing brain lesions. TGA never was actually diagnosed in this patient but in retrospect it was the most tenable diagnosis. His manifestations and repetitive questioning were classical for this condition.

As mentioned, the well-known vasospastic component of migraine so closely parallels the strongly suspected vasospastic component of transient global amnesia, many researchers suspect a close relationship between the two conditions.[28-36] Some insist that all classic transient global amnesia cases are reflections of an underlying migraine process, regardless of the history. Migraine headaches are extremely common and characteristically one-sided, at least at the start. Not all headaches of unilateral presentation have the so-called premonitory visual aura. Indeed the aura associated 'classic' migraine is seen much less frequently than common migraine. Many common migraine patients report a foreboding awareness of a headache "to come," some time before the pain begins. Others demonstrate a subtle personality change that heralds to both patients and observers alike that a headache is about to begin. On the other hand, visual aura frequently is not followed by headache, even those auras having subjectively very prominent visual aberrations. The judgment of many authorities is that aura represent a form of "spreading reaction" in the visual cortex and as such has a neurophysiological relationship to the presumed spreading reaction of transient global amnesia, where the brain areas involved are the memory processing areas.

As I mentioned briefly in Chapter I, Oliver Sacks, in his book, *The Man Who Mistook His Wife for a Hat*,"[37] gives us an unforgettable picture of Jimmie, a serious alcoholic in his younger years, whose resulting permanent memory loss from the chronic effects of alcoholism forever locked him in his Navy years of the early forties "with Truman at the helm." This man, with remarkable ease, could somehow relate all new technology, even progress in space flight, comfortably back to his WW2 years but could retain no specific event after 1945. He never admitted any new events that did not fit his world. Moreover, in this remarkable example of permanent global amnesia, Sacks' every visit to his unfortunate patient during more than a decade of follow-up was like the first visit--Jimmie was never able to recall he had met this impressive doctor dozens of times before. Sacks describes transient global amnesia as an acute (and mercifully transient) Korsakoff's syndrome. He recalled a case, revealed to him by an associate, involving a highly intelligent man who, for a period of some hours, was unable to remember his wife and children or even that he had a wife and children. In effect, this man had lost thirty years of his life though, fortunately, for only the few hours that his global amnesia lasted. Sacks sees such events as most horrifying in their power to absolutely annul or obliterate decades of richly lived, richly achieved and richly remembered life.

Sacks continues in his uniquely eloquent style to say that only others, typically, feel the horror. The patient is unaware, amnesiac for his amnesia, and only later learns that, for a day, he had lost half a lifetime and never knew it. These short-lived amnesia cases associated with early-onset Korsakoff's syndrome can easily be confused with classic transient global amnesia.

The literature reports a number of cases of infectious disease of the central nervous system presenting first as transient global amnesia.[38-39] Even before the more telltale symptoms and signs of headache, febrile response, nuchal rigidity and stupor develop, transient global amnesia may herald the onset of meningo-encephalitis. Both the herpes simplex and Epstein-Barr virus have presented as classical transient global amnesia, thus underscoring the need to suspect a possibly infectious origin, regardless of the age of the patient and absence of the more usual signs of infection.

Although hypoglycemia usually presents with the more characteristic symptoms of irritability, tiredness, confusion and mood changes, other occasionally encountered symptoms of altered responsiveness, forgetfulness and inattention frequently suggest the diagnosis of transient global amnesia. We were told of the painful reality of a young doctor in a clinic who was the unfortunate victim of hypoglycemic attacks. Almost always, these presented with a rapidly progressive paucity of motion and facial expression that transformed him into a quiet, slow motion version of his former self. Predictably, patient reaction was guarded at the sight of the doctor who, only moments before had been normal in all respects, now appeared nearly frozen in time. Minutes after Glucagon injection, expression and animation rapidly returned. The doctor would once again "return" to the scene, intent on resuming his task of taking a blood pressure or applying his stethoscope to a patient's lung fields. He was totally oblivious that perhaps ten minutes had passed and he could not understand the fact that the patient had long since departed. During this time period, despite being awake and apparently alert, nothing registered with him and anterograde amnesia was complete. One could only wonder if his transition from the functional to non-functional state was instantaneous and hope, out of compassion for the young doctor, that it was, for in this event he could do little harm other than to patient confidence. However, professional experience suggests otherwise for he must have been semi-functional at times, the worse case scenario for a doctor. Somehow, in his four years of medical school and one year of internship this disability had not been filtered out.

Other cases of altered responsiveness and amnesia are occasionally seen with certain prescription medications, such as the sedatives and hypnotics drugs of the benzodiazapine class. The temporary memory impairment may be quite similar to that of transient global amnesia.[40-44] Triazolam, one of the shorter acting benzodiazapines promoted for use as a hypnotic, has become quite notorious as the culprit in traveler's amnesia. Frequently, these lapses have been associated with ethanol ingestion, but a surprising number of reports cite a transient global amnesia syndrome resulting from the ingestion of a single oral dose of other benzodiazapines. This was also true of the even the longer acting lorazapam and diazapam.

This subject will no doubt be of considerable interest and concern to military doctors and flight surgeons. In their effort to help troops being rapidly deployed to other parts of the world adjust their day/night cycle and prevent jetlag, they are charged with the responsibility of administering benzodiazapine drugs such as triazolam. The obvious purpose is to help ensure that troops arrive at their destination as rested as possible, free of jet lag and fully functional. Temporary memory impairment of some individuals is one of the unavoidable risks of large-scale use of these drugs.

Memory disturbance closely resembling transient global amnesia has been commonly reported with alcohol and marijuana intoxication as well as with use of the drug known as clioquinol.[45-46] They differ only in that the duration of the amnesia may last for several days and be associated with a permanent retrograde amnesia extending back weeks and months. Because patient history in such cases of amnesia is irrelevant, in the absence of observer history the diagnosis of drug intoxication may be confused with transient global amnesia. The literature is replete with descriptions of the "blackout spells" associated with alcoholic bouts but rarely, if ever, would these obviously sensory- impaired cases be mistaken for the alert, articulate and disarmingly functional transient global amnesia patient. Chronic alcoholism is not always obvious to the busy emergency room examiner.

A Holocaust survivor who developed sudden amnesia during a subsequent psychiatric intake interview[47] clearly demonstrated the ability of repressed memories to trigger an amnesic "escape from reality" remarkably similar to classic transient global amnesia.

Another example is the remarkable case history of the 'Nowhere Man" in the Evansville Courier Express.[48] Helen O'Neill, an AP special correspondent, presented the pathetic tale of a man in his late twenties with a distinctive British accent who awoke in a hospital in November of 1999. He did not know who he was or where he came from. The man's photograph and fingerprints were circulated around the world and television programs documented his plight. Interpol and international missing persons organizations investigated. Doctors and psychologists and detectives probed. Now, nearly three years later, there are still no leads as to the origin of the "Nowhere Man." Predictably, without a birth date, name, social security number or passport, this man is trapped in a state of limbo. No one who has dealt with him doubts his story. He has found some clues about himself--that he loves to read, that he took milk and sugar with his tea and that he didn't like meat. No one has claimed him. No one knows him. He is singularly alone. Psychiatrist called into his case feel he has escaped from memories too awful to remember into his present, non-existent status.

Roman-Campos[49] reported a 64-year old woman who had an unusual, transient global amnesia state with anterograde memory loss for ten days and a permanent retrograde loss of between five to ten years of her life. The patient had no neurologic signs during the episode and recovered completely. The EEG suggested a left medial temporal lobe area of dysfunction. One may infer from this that the distinction between a protracted transient global amnesia case such as this and a prolonged psychogenic fugue state is not always clear.

Presented with this list of "differential diagnostic possibilities," to use the traditional medical jargon, it is not easy to make the diagnosis of classic transient global amnesia with complete assurance. The stumbling blocks to accurate diagnosis are many. Even the imaging studies done as part of the usual emergency room evaluation, although reasonably definitive for CVA and space occupying lesion, would be of little help with a new amnestic seizure patient or subtle head trauma case wherein all reasonable diagnostic studies might be negative. Despite these confounding possibilities, the literature now contains reports of well over 1,000 cases of transient global amnesia since Bender's index case of 1956. On this basis, one could calculate an average incidence of about 20 cases per year. Clearly many factors other than statin drugs have made their contribution over the years but the recent surge in transient global amnesia cases associated with statin drug use [50] is a sobering observation.

This is all the more worrisome as the pharmaceutical industry plans for expanded use of these drugs, even for children.

* * *

REFERENCES

CHAPTER I – Lipitor,® Thief of Memory
1. Sacks O. *The Man Who Mistook His Wife For A Hat.* Summit Books, 1985.
2. Ibid.
3. Keys A. Coronary heart disease in seven countries. *Circulation* 41, Supplement 1, 1970.

CHAPTER II- What is Transient Global Amnesia?
1. Bender MB. Syndrome of isolated episode of confusion with amnesia. *Journal of the Hillside Hospital* 5, 212-215, 1956.
2. Hodges JR, Warlow CP. The aetiology of transient global amnesia: A case-control study of 114 cases with prospective follow-up. *Brain* 113, 639-657, 1990.
3. Litch JA, Bishop RA. Transient global amnesia at high altitude. *New England Journal of Medicine* 340, 1444, 1999.
4. Simons J. PFIZER, The $10 Billion Pill," *Fortune,* 6 January, 2003.
5. Pfrieger F. Brain Researcher Discovers Bright Side of Ill-Famed Molecule. *Science,* 9 November, 2001.
6. Golomb B and others. Amnesia in Association with Statin Use. UCSD College of Medicine, Statin Research Study, 2002 (under review).
7. Wagstaff LR and others. Statin-associated memory loss: analysis of 60 case reports and review of the literature. *Pharmacotherapy 23(7),* 871-880, 2003.

CHAPTER III -The Formation of Memory and Its Transformation in TGA
1. Kandel ER. *Cellular Mechanism of Learning and the biological basis of individuality.* Principles of Neural Science, New York, Elsevier, 1985.
2. Tully T and others. Genetic dissection of consolidated memory in Drosophila. *Cell* 79, 39-47, 1994.
3. Silva AJ and others. Gene targeting and the biology of learning and memory. *Annual Review of Genetics* 31, 527-546, 1997.
4. Ridley M. *Genome, The Autobiography of a Species in 23 Chapters.* Harper Collins, 2000.
5. Davis RL. Mushroom Bodies and Drosophila, *Neurone* 11, 1-14, 1993.
6. Grotewiel MS and others. Integrin-mediated short-term memory in Drosophila, *Nature* 391, 455-460, 1998.

7.   Pfrieger F. Brain Researcher Discovers Bright Side of Ill-Famed Molecule. *Science*, 9 November, 2001.
8.   Brousseau ME, Schaefer, EJ,."Structure and mechanism of action of HMG-CoA reductase inhibitors "in *HMG-CoA Reductase Inhibitors,* Schmitz, G., Torzewski, M, Eds., Basel, Schweiz, Birkhauser, 2002.
9.   Wagstaff LR and others. Statin-associated memory loss: analysis of 60 case reports and review of the literature. *Pharmacotherapy 23(7)*, 871-880, 2003.
10.   Schwartz G and others. Effects of Atorvastatin on early recurrent ischemic events in acute coronary syndromes. *Journal of the American Medical Association* 285 (13), 1711-1717, 2002.
11.   Sever PS and others. Prevention of Coronary and Stoke Events With Atorvastatin In Hypertensive Patients Who Have Average Or Lower-Than Average Cholesterol Concentrations in the Anglo-Scandinavian Cardiac Outcomes Trial. *Lancet 361,* 1149-1158, 2003.
12.   The Allhat Officers and Coordinators For the Allhat Collaborative Research Group. Major Outcomes In Moderately Hypercholesterolemic, Hypertensive Patients Randomized to Pravastatin vs. Usual Care: The Antihypertensive and Lipid Lowering Treatment To Prevent Heart Attack Trial. *Journal of the American Medical Association 288,* 2998-3007, 2002.
13.   Collins R and others. Heart Protection Study of Cholesterol Lowering With Simvastatin in 5963 People With Diabetes. *Lancet* 361, 2005-2016, 2003.
14.   Ravnskov U. *The Cholesterol Myths*, NewTrends Publishing, 2000.
15.   Cohen JS. *Over Dose, The Case Against the Pharmaceutical Companies*, Tarcher/Putnam, 2001

CHAPTER IV - How the Statin Drugs Work

1.   Heber D and others. Cholesterol lowering effects of a proprietary Chinese red yeast rice dietary supplement. *American Journal of Clinical Nutrition 69,* 231-236, 1999.
2.   Folkers K and others. Lovastatin decreases Coenzyme Q levels in humans, *Proceedings of the National. Academy of Sciences 87.* 8931-8934, 1990.
3.   Langsjoen P, Langsjoen A. Coenzyme Q10 In cardiovascular disease with emphasis on heart failure and myocardial ischemia. *Asia Pacific Heart Journal* 7(3), 160-168, 1998.

4.   Langsjoen P, Langsjoen A. Statin associated congestive heart failure. *Proceedings of Weston-Price Foundation Meeting,* Spring, 2003.
5.   Gaist D and others. Statins and the risk of polyneuropathy: A case control study. *Neurology* 58, 1333-1337, 2002.
6.   Sparks S. Written personal communication. 8 August, 2003.
7.   Golomb B and others. Amnesia in Association with Statin Use. UCSD College of Medicine, Statin Research Study, 2002 (under review).
8.   Wolfe S. Public Citizen Petitions FDA To Warn Doctors, Patients About Cholesterol Drugs, 20 August, 2001.
9.   Whitaker J. Citizens' Petition filed with FDA:to include Coenzyme Q10 use recommendation in all statin drug labeling. *Life Extension Magazine,* May 23, 2002.
10.   Griffiths G, Simons K. The Trans-Golgi Network: Sorting at the Exit Side of the Golgi Complex, *Science 243,* 438-442, 1986.
11.   DNAprint Genomics, http://www.dnaprint.com.

CHAPTER V - The Role of Cholesterol in the Body

1.   Guyton AC, Hall JE. *The Adrenocortical Hormones.* In *Textbook of Medical Physiology, 9th Ed,* 957-971, Saunders, Philadelphia, 1996.
2.   Russel DW. Green Light for Steroid Hormones. *Science 272,* 370-371, 1996.
3.   Pfrieger F. Brain Researcher Discovers Bright Side of Ill-Famed Molecule. *Science,* 9 November, 2001.
4.   Ibid.
5.   Muldoon MF and others. Cholesterol Reduction and Non-Illness Mortality. Meta-Analysis of Randomized Clinical Trials. *British Medical Journal* 322, 11-15, 2001.
6.   Golomb BA. Cholesterol and Violence: Is There a Connection? *Annals of Internal Medicine 128,* 478-487, 1998.
7.   Wolozin B and others. Decreased Prevalence of Alzheimer Disease Associated With 3-Hydroxy-3-Methyglutaryl Coenzyme A Reduction Inhibitors. *Archives of Neurology* 57, 1439-1443, 2000.
8.   Golomb B. Statins and Dementia. *Letters to the Editor, Archives of Neurology 58(7),* July 2001.
9.   Kaplan M. Low Cholesterol Causes Aggressive Behavior and Depression. *Psychosomatic Medicine* 56, 479-484, 1994.
10.   Bender KJ. *Psychiatric Times 15(5),* 1998.
11.   Duits N, Bos F. Depressive Symptoms and Cholesterol Lowering Drugs. *Lancet* 341, Letter, 1999

12. Lechleitner M. Depressive Symptoms in Hypercholesterolaemic Patients Treated With Pravastatin. *Lancet* 340, Letter, 1999.
13. Buydens-Branchey L, Branchey M. Association between low plasma levels of cholesterol and relapse in cocaine addicts. *Psychosomatic Medicine* 65, 86-91, 2003.
14. Horwich TB and others. Low Serum total cholesterol is associated with marked increase in mortality in advanced heart failure. *Journal of Cardiac Failure 8(4)*, 2002.
15. McCully KS. *The Homocysteine Revolution*. Keats, 1997

CHAPTER VI - The Arteriosclerosis, Cholesterol, Homocysteine Connection

1. McCully KS. *The Homocysteine Revolution*. Keats, 1997
2. Ibid.
3. Ibid
4. McCully K. Homocysteine theory of arteriosclerosis: Development and current status. In Gotto AM, Paolett R., editors, *Atherosclerosis Reviews* 11, 157-246, Raven Press, New York, 1983.
5. McCully K. Atherosclerosis, serum cholesterol and the homocysteine theory: A study of 194 consecutive autopsies. *.American Journal of the American Sciences* 299, 217-221, 1990.
6. McCully KS. *The Homocysteine Revolution*, Keats, 1997
7. Brown MS, Goldstein JL. Expression of the familial hypercholesterolemia gene in heterozygotes: Mechanism for a dominant disorder in man. *Science* 185, 61-63, 1974.
8. McCully KS. *The Homocysteine Revolution*. Keats, 1997.
9. Ibid.
10. Wilcken DE, Wilcken B. The pathogenesis of coronary heart disease. A possible role for methionine metabolism. *Journal of Clinical Investigation* 57,1079-1082, 1976.
11. Boushey CJ and others. A quantitative assessment of plasma homocysteine as a risk factor for vascular disease. *Journal of the American Medical Association* 274, 1049-1057, 1995.
12. Kannel WB. The role of cholesterol in coronary atherogenesis. *Medical clinics of North America* 58, 363-379, 1974.
13. Kauffman J. Should you take aspirin to prevent heart attack? *Journal of Scientific Exploration* 14 (4), 623-641, 2000.
14. Collins R. Statin Drug Study of Patients at High Risk For Heart Disease. *Oxford University, American Heart Association*, 2001.
15. Golomb B and others. Amnesia in Association with Statin Use. UCSD College of Medicine, Statin Research Study, 2002 (under review).

16. Ravnskov U. *The Cholesterol Myths*, NewTrends Publishing, 2000.
17. Ottoboni A, Ottoboni F. *The Modern Nutritional Diseases*. Vincente Books, Inc., Sparks, NV, 2002.
18. Kauffman J. Should you take aspirin to prevent heart attack? *Journal of Scientific Exploration* 14 (4), 623-641, 2000.

CHAPTER VII - The Myth of the Cholesterol/Modified Low Fat Diet
1. Atkins, R. Dr. *Atkins' New Diet Revolution*. 3rd Edit, Evans, New York, 2002.
2. Taubes G. What If It's All Been A Big, Fat Lie? *New York Times Magazine*, July 7, 2002.
3 Eades MR, Eades MD. *Protein Power*. Bantam Books, 1996.
4. Sears B. *The Zone*. Harper Collins, 1997.
5. Steward H and others. *Sugar Busters*. Ballentine Books, 1998.
6. McCully KS, McCully M. *The Heart Revolution*. Harper Collins, 2000.
7. Willett W. Turning The Food Pyramid Up Side Down. *American Journal of Clinical Nutrition 76,1261-1271,* 2002.
8. Taubes G. What If It's All Been A Big, Fat Lie? *New York Times Magazine*, July 7, 2002.
9. Enig MG, Fallon S. The Mediterranean Diet--Pasta or Pastrami? *The Weston A..Price Foundation Magazine,* Spring, 2000.
10. Keys A. Coronary heart disease in seven countries, *Circulation 41(supplement 1)*, 1970.
11. Ibid.
12. Ravnskov U. *The Cholesterol Myths*, NewTrends Publishing, 2000.
13. Foster-Powell K and others. International "Table of Glycemic Index and Glycemic Load Values. *American Journal of Clinical Nutrition* 76, 5-56, 2002.
14. Taubes G. What If It's All Been A Big, Fat Lie? *New York Times Magazine*, July 7, 2002.
15. Ibid.

CHAPTER VIII - What Diet, Then? Rethinking the Food Pyramid
1. McCully KS, McCully M. *The Heart Revolution*. Harper Collins, 2000.
2. Ibid.
3. Atkins RC. *Dr.Atkins' New Diet Revolution*. Evans, New York, 2002.

4.   Kauffman J. Low Carbohydrate Diets. *Journal of Scientific Exploration,* 2004. (under review)
5.   Braly J, Hoggan R. *Dangerous Grains: Why Gluten Cereal May Be Hazardous To Your Health.* Avery/Penguin Putnam, New York, 2002.
6.   Ottoboni A, Ottoboni F. *The Modern Nutritional Diseases: Heart Disease, Stroke, Type-2 Diabetes, Obesity, Cancer, and How To Prevent Them.* Vincenti Books, Sparks, NV, 2002.
7.   McCully KS, McCully M. *The Heart Revolution.* Harper Collins, 2000.
8.   Bernstein, R. *Dr. Bernstein's Diabetes Solution.* Little, Brown, Boston, 1997.
9.   Smith MD. *Going Against the Grain: How Reducing and Avoiding Grains Can Revitalize Your Health.* Contemporary Books, Chicago, 2002.
10.   Allan C, Lutz W. *Life Without Bread: How a Low-Carbohydrate Diet Can Save Your Life.* Keats, Los Angeles, 2000.
11.   Groves B. *Eat Fat Get Thin.* Vermilion, London, 1999.
12.   Eades MR, Eades MD. *The Protein Power Lifeplan.* Warner Books, New York, 2000.
13.   Atkins RC. *Dr.Atkins' New Diet Revolution.* Evans, New York, 2002.
14.   Kwasniewski MD, Chylinski M. *Homo Optimus.* Wydawnictwo WGP, Warsaw, 2000
15.   Enig M, Fallon S. The Oiling of America. *Nexus Magazine,* Feb-Mar, 1999.
16.   McCully KS, McCully M. *The Heart Revolution.* Harper Collins, 2000.
17.   Fallon S, Enig M. What causes heart disease? *Lancet* 1,: 1062-1065, 1983
18.   Kauffman J. Should you take aspirin to prevent heart attack? *Journal of Scientific Exploration* 14 (4), 623-641, 2000.
19.   McCully KS, McCully M. *The Heart Revolution.* Harper Collins, 2000.

CONCLUSION

1.   McCully KS. *The Homocysteine Revolution.* Keats, 1997.
2.   Pfrieger F. Brain Researcher Discovers Bright Side of Ill-Famed Molecule. *Science,* 9 November, 2001.
3.   Golomb B and others. Amnesia in Association with Statin Use. UCSD College of Medicine, Statin Research Study, 2002 (under review).

4.   Cohen JS. *Over Dose, The Case Against the Pharmaceutical Companies*, Tarcher/Putnam, 2001
5.   Allred J. Lowering Serum Cholesterol: Who Benefits? 1993, *Journal of Nutrition* 123: 1453-1459, 1993.
6.   McCully KS, McCully M. *The Heart Revolution*. Harper Collins, 2000.
7.   Lee KW, Lip GYH. The Role of Omega-3 in the Secondary Prevention of Cardiovascular Disease. *Quarterly Journal of Medicine* 96, 465-480, 2003.
8.   Langsjoen PH, Langsjoen AM. Overview Of The Use of Coenzyme In Cardiovascular Disease. *Cardiovascular Disease Biofactors 9*, (Issue 2-4), 273-285, 1999.
9.   Kauffman J. Should you take aspirin to prevent heart attack? *Journal of Scientific Exploration* 14 (4), 623-641, 2000.
12.   Collins R. Statin Drug Study of Patients at High Risk For Heart Disease. *Oxford University, American Heart Association*, 2001.
13.   Jackson PR and others. Statins for primary prevention: At what coronary risk is safety assured? *British Journal of Clinical Pharmacology* 52, 439-446, 2001.
14.   Schwartz GG and others. Effects of Atorvastatin on Early Recurrent Ischemic Events in Acute Coronary Syndromes. *Journal of American Medical Association* 285, 1711-1718, 2001.
13.   Simons J. PFIZER, The $10 Billion Pill. *Fortune*, 6 January 2003.
16.   Cohen JS. *Over Dose, The Case Against the Pharmaceutical Companies*, Tarcher/Putnam, 2001.

ADDENDUM-Part I - Mechanisms of Action of Transient Global Amnesia

1.   Lewis SL. Aetiology of Transient Global Amnesia. *Lancet* 352, 9125,1998.
2.   Homma S. PFO in cryptogenic stroke study. *Circulation* 105(22), 2625, 2002.
3.   Richter F. Migraine aura and spreading depression. *Annals of Neurology 49 7-13,* 2001.
4.   Pfrieger F. Brain Researcher Discovers Bright Side of Ill-Famed Molecule. *Science*, 9 November, 2001.

ADDENDUM-Part II - Differential Diagnosis of Transient Global Amnesia

1.   Vohanka S, Zouhar A. Transient global amnesia after mild head injury in childhood. *Act Nerv Super* (Praha) 30 (1), 68-74, 1988.

2.   Haas DC, Ross GS. Transient global amnesia triggered by mild head trauma. *Brain* 109 (2), 251-257, 1986.

3.   Heckl RW, Baum R. Episodes of amnesia following whiplash injury to the cervical spine. *Aktuelle Traumatol* 14(1), 33-36, 1984.

4.   Schacter DL. *Searching for Memory*, Basic Books, 1996.

5.   Palmini Al and others. Pure amnestic epilepsy. Definition, clinical symptomatology and functional anatomical considerations. *Brain* 115 (3), 749-769, 1992.

6.   Stracciari A and others. Epileptic transient amnesia. *Eur Neurol* 30(3), 176-179, 1990.

7.   Tassinari CA and others. Transient global amnesia as a postictal state from recurrent partial seizures. *Epilepsia* 32(6), 882-885, 1991.

8.   Cole AJ and others. Transient global amnesia: the electroencephalogram at onset. *Annals of Neurology* 22(6), 771-772, 1987.

9.   Dugan TM and others. Transient global amnesia associated with bradycardia and temporal lobe spikes. *Cortex* 17(4), 633-637, 1981.

10.   Gallassi R and others. Epileptic transient amnesia. *Italian Journal of Neurological Science supplement 9,* 37-39, 1988.

11.   Galllassi R and others. Epileptic amnesic syndrome., *Epilepsia* 33, supplement 6, 521-525, 1992.

12.   Richard P, Brenner RP. Absence Status. Case Reports and a review of the literature. *Encephale* 6(4), 385-392, 1980.

13.   Shuping JR and others. Transient global amnesia due to glioma in the dominant hemisphere. *Neurology* 30(1), 88-90, 1980.

14.   Stracciari A and others. Transient global amnesia associated with a large arachnoid cyst of the middle cranial fossa of the non dominant hemisphere. *Italian Journal of Neurological Science* 8(6), 609-611, 1987.

15.   Araga S and others. Transient global amnesia and falcotentorial meningioma-a case report. *Japanese Journal of Psychiatry and Neurology* 43(2), 201-203, 1989.

16.   Arnetoli G and others. Permanent amnesia as a result of a bilateral lesion of the hippocampus: description of a clinical case. *Riv Patol Nerv Ment* 104(4), 151-157, 1983.

17.   Boudin G and others. Glioma of the posterior limbic system revealed by transient global amnesia. Anatomic-clinical observations of one case. *Rev Neurol* (Paris)131(3), 157-163, 1975.

18. Cattaino G.and others. Ethmoidal meningioma revealed by transient global amnesia. *Italian Journal of Neurological Science* 10(2), 187-191, 1989.

19. Findler G and others. Transient global amnesia associated with a single metastasis in the non-dominant hemisphere. Case report. *Journal of Neurosurgery* 58(2), 303-305, 1983.

20. Honda M and others. P300 abnormalities in patients with selective impairment of recent memory. *Journal of Neurological Science* 139(1), 95-105, 1996.

21. Honma Y, Nagao S. Hemorrhagic pituitary adenoma manifesting as transient global amnesia. *Neurol Med Chir* (Tokyo) 36(4), 234-236, 1996.

22. Bogousslavsky J, Regli F. Transient global amnesia and stroke. *Eur Neurol* 28(2), 106-110, 1988.

23. Goldenberg G and others. Amnesic syndrome with a unilateral thalamic lesion: a case report. *Journal of Neurology* 229(2), 79-86, 1983.

24. Gorelick PB and others. Transient global amnesia and thalamic infarction. *Neurology* 38(3), 496-499, 1998.

25. Greer DM and others. Unilateral temporal lobe stroke causing ischemic transient global amnesia: a role for diffusion-weighted imaging in the initial evaluation. *Journal of Neuroimaging*, 2001.

26. Jacome DE. EEG features in transient global amnesia. *Clinical Electroencephalography* 20(3), 183-192, 1989.

27. Takahashi Y and others. Transient global amnesia and dural arteriovenous fistula of the anterior cranial fossa. *Kurume Medical Journal* 43(3), 223-229, 1996.

28. Pradalier A and others. Transient global amnesia, migraine, thalamic infarct, dihydroergotamine, and sumatriptan. *Headache*, 2000.

29. Guidotti M and others. A case-control study of transient global amnesia. *Journal Neurology and Neurosurgical Psychiatry* 52(3), 320-323, 1989.

30. Jensen TS, De Fine Olivarius B. Transient global amnesia as a manifestation of transient cerebral ischemia. *Acta Neurol Scan* 61(2), 115-124, 1980.

31. Santos S and others. Transient global amnesia: a review of 58 cases. *Rev Neurol* 30, 1113-1117, 2000.

32. Attarian S and others. A case of transient amnesia caused by cerebral thrombophlebitis: contribution of neuroimaging to physiopathogenesis of transient amnesia. *Rev Neurol* (Paris)151(10),.552-558, 1995.

33. Ay H and others. Diffusion-weighted MRI characterizes the ischemic lesion in transient global amnesia. *Neurology* 51(3), 901-903, 1998.

34. Chen ST and others. Transient global amnesia and amaurosis fugax in a patient with common carotid artery occlusion-a case report. *Angiology* 51(3), 257-261, 2000.

35. Chen WH and others. Transient global amnesia and thalamic hemorrhage. *Clinical Journal of Neurology and Neurosurgery* 98(4), 309-311, 1996.

36. Chatham PE, Brillman J. Transient global amnesia associated with bilateral subdural hematomas. *Neurosurgery* 17(6), 971-973, 1985.

37. Sacks O. *The Man Who Mistook His Wife For A Hat.* Summit Books, 1985.

38. Mizutani T and others Unusual neurologic manifestations associated with Epstein-Barr virus infection. *Internal Medicine* 32(1), 36-38, 1993.

39. Pommer B and others. Transient global amnesia as a manifestation of Epstein-Barr virus encephalitis. *Journal of Neurology* 229(2), 125-127, 1983.

40. Morris HH III, Estes ML. Traveler's amnesia. Transient global amnesia secondary to triazolam. *Journal of the American Medical Asso*ciation 258(7), 945-946, 1987.

41. Regard M, Landis T. Transient global amnesia: neuropsychological dysfunction during attack and recover in two "pure" cases." Journal of Neurology and Neurosurgical Psychiatry 47(7), 668-672, 1984.

42. Seifert D and others. Midazolam-a forensic problem drug? *Blutalkohol* 27(5), 326-331, 1990.

43. Vinson DC. Acute transient memory loss. *American Family Physician* 39(5), 249-254, 1989.

44. Kohase HF and others. Transient Global Amnesia after generalized anesthesia. *Masui* 47(4), 481-483, 1998.

45. Mumenthaler M and others. Transient global amnesia after clioquinol: five personal observations from outside Japan. *Journal of Neurology and Neurosurgical Psychiatry* 42(12), 1084-1089, 1979.

46. Kaeser HE. Transient global amnesia due to clioquionol. *Acta Neuro Scand Supplement* 100, 175-183, 1984.

47. Durst R and others. Amnestic state in a Holocaust survivor patient: psychogenic versus neurological basis. *Isr Journal Psychiatry Relat Sci* 36(1), 47-54, 1999.

48. O'Neill H. Nowhere Man. *Evansville Courier Express,* 22 October, 2001.

49.   Roman-Campos G and others. Persistent retrograde memory deficit after transient global amnesia. *Cortex* 16(3), 509-518, 1980.

GLOSSARY

Aldosterone - *one of a group of hormones produced by the adrenal gland that has a primary role in maintaining salt and water balance in the body.*

Alpha integrin - *a biologic "glue" with the function of binding synaptic connections that are involved in memory.*

Amino acids - *DNA derived nitrogen-containing organic compounds that are essential components of protein. Protein, when metabolized, breaks down into its various amino acids.*

Amnesiac - *a person who is having, or has had, amnesia. Also the adjective form of the noun amnesia, i.e., someone who is amnesiac for an event.*

Amnestic - *resembling amnesia.*

Androgen - *a hormone that develops and maintains masculine characteristics.*

Aneurysm - *a swelling of the wall of a blood vessel that is usually due to some inherent or acquired weakness. In some cases an aneurysm may develop in a healthy vessel simply because the pressure within is excessive.*

Angiography - *the procedure of injecting a radio-opaque dye into the blood vessel, or in some cases lymphatic vessels, to delineate their internal configuration.*

Aphasia - *the loss of the ability to express and understand ideas, usually in response to some brain disease.*

Apraxia - *the loss of ability to execute or carry out familiar (previously learned) movements.*

Arteriosclerosis - *the progressive thickening and hardening of the wall of an artery with deposition of fibrotic strands and calcium accumulation. The inside of the artery, known as the lumen, may become progressively* reduced, leading to diminished blood flow. *Many factors are involved in this process including blood pressure and various genetic and nutritional deficiencies.*

Bile acid sequestrants - *these sequestrants, using an ionic exchange principle, bind the bile acids derived from cholesterol as they are secreted into the intestine by the liver, thereby allowing their excretion.*

Black Box Warning - *the extreme toxicity warning the FDA requires pharmaceutical companies to include in the prescription information furnished to doctors in package inserts and in the Physicians Desk Reference (PDR).*

Blood brain barrier - *the term used to describe a relative barrier to chemical substances in the blood based on the molecular size and configuration of the chemical involved. Small chemical complexes pass readily into the brain but large complexes, such as the well-known LDL complex of protein and cholesterol, cannot pass.*

Calcitrol - *a hormone produced from cholesterol which has primary control of the calcium balance within the body.*

Cardiomyopathy - *inflammation of the heart muscle.*

Cerebral edema - *swelling of the brain.*

Cerivastatin - *the generic name for Baycol.*

Cognitive - *those brain functions that have to do with memory in one form or another. From simple forgetfulness, confusion and disorientation, the spectrum of cognitive effects may extend to the complete obliteration of memory in a condition know as amnesia. This loss of cognitive function may be patchy, vague and transient.*

Cortical - *referring to the outer, gray layer of the brain known as the cortex.*

CPK - *creatine phosphokinase, an enzyme released into the blood stream by inflamed muscle tissue.*

CREB - *cyclic response element binding, the protein that is intimately involved in the formation and retention of memory.*

CRP - *C-reactive protein, a non-specific test for inflammation in the body.*

Cyclic AMP - *cyclic adenosine mono-phosphate, a part of the energy reservoir of the body that is intimately involved in the process of memory formation.*

Dementia - *the loss of intellectual capacities usually associated with profound emotional changes.*

Diabesity - *a recent term referring to the increasingly frequent presence of a combination of obesity and type 2 diabetes in both adults and children.*

Diabetes type 2 - *the so-called "adult onset diabetes" representing an exhaustion of the insulin producing capacity of the pancreas, due to excessive carbohydrate stimulation. The condition is relative and is occasionally responsive to oral medication designed to stimulate more insulin production but is more effectively treated by an aggressive carbohydrate-restrictive diet.*

Dinoflagellate toxicity - *a marine protozoan occasionally infecting fish or other marine creatures and producing a chemical which causes unusual cognitive side effects (among other symptoms) in humans exposed to the chemical.*

Dolichols - *a class of chemical that play a key role in the transfer of information within a cell. These chemicals help "package" messages to transmitter proteins, thereby insuring that messages reach their proper target within the cell.*

Estrogen - *a hormone produced primarily in the ovaries and responsible, in part for the reproductive process and the development and maintenance of feminine characteristics.*

Fibric acid derivative - *a class of lipid lowering chemicals especially effective on the fraction of lipids known as triglycerides, and transported by the very low density protein carriers. The precise mechanism of action has never been definitively established.*

Flashback - *the occasional occurrence of symptoms of a drug's side effects happening long after the drug has been discontinued and has presumably left the body.*

Fluvastatin - *the generic name for Lescol.*

Gastrectomy - *removal of part or all of the stomach, formerly a common procedure done in the presence of severe gastritis and ulcers resistant to other available forms of treatment. Current knowledge determines that a these conditions are caused by a certain class of bacteria and are best treated with antibiotics.*

Glial cells - *cells within the brain which have a maintenance and repair function. They are the primary source of brain cell cholesterol without which transmission of information within the brain would be impossible.*

Hemorrhagic stroke - *stroke caused by the rupture of an artery previously weakened by disease. Occasionally, it is present with poor blood clotting or excessive levels of the commonly used drug, coumadin.*

Hydrophilic - *a term meaning "water loving," reflecting the tendency for certain chemicals to be soluble in water.*

Hypercholesterolemia - *the condition of excessively high cholesterol levels in the body. The standards defining high or elevated cholesterol are constantly being changed, depending upon evolving treatment philosophies and options. Current medicines available can result in dramatic decreases in serum cholesterol, even as the true role of cholesterol in the human body is beginning to be defined and appreciated.*

Hypoglycemia - *low blood glucose, occasionally the cause of dramatic and severe body reactions including memory dysfunction. At one time, hypoglycemia induced by insulin injections under controlled conditions was used to trigger seizures in the treatment of severe depression.*

Ischemic - *poor blood supply to an area, usually due to some form of blockage of the perfusing artery or other means of curtailing blood flow.*

Ketosis high - *a feeling of exhilaration sometimes experienced when metabolizing mostly body fat to supply energy needs. It is the result of a kind of "starvation" metabolism that results in a build-up within the body of ketones, the end products of fat metabolism.*

Korsakoff's syndrome - *a condition seen in chronic alcoholics wherein a permanent memory loss occurs for which the pathetic victim often attempts to compensate by "making up" memory to fill the gaps.*

Lipids - *a general term for all the various types of fats that make up the body.*

Lipophilic - *the term means "fat-loving" and reflects a tendency for some chemicals to be soluble in fats rather than water. Such chemicals are taken up more avidly by the human brain.*

Lipoprotein - *the chemical complex that results when cholesterol and other lipids such as triglycerides combine with a protein carrier in order to be transported freely in the body.*

Lovastatin - *the generic name for Mevacor.*

Low-pressure chamber - *a device used primarily by aerospace researcher and industries to simulate various altitudes. For example, jet pilots must "ascend" to 25,000 and 35,000 feet equivalent altitude in these chambers in order to train in oxygen mask use. Such training usually involves "masks off" demonstrations at these altitudes so that each pilot or flight crewmember can learn their personal reaction to oxygen deprivation. These chambers are also used to simulate rapid decompression emergencies at altitude and even "free fall from 50,000 to 100,000 feet equivalent to simulate emergency ejection and parachute descent.*

Macrophage - *cells of various types within our bodies which have the function of engulfing and digesting foreign material such as bacteria and viruses and thereby ridding the body of them.*

Medial temporal - *a medical reference term used to describe the location of something located on the inner aspect of the temporal lobes of the brain, an area deep within the brain.*

Mitochondria - *tiny storehouses of energy within each of our cells. From an evolutionary viewpoint, these structures may at one time have been separate free-living organisms.*

Monocyte - *one of several types of white blood cells with the ability to function as a macrophage in fighting infection or inflammation in the body.*

Morbidity rate - *term used to describe the prevalence of a condition such as heart disease, hypertension, and usually expressed as numbers (cases) per unit of time.*

Mortality rate - *term used to describe the number of deaths per unit of time; for example, heart attack deaths per month.*

MRI - *magnetic resonance imaging. One of many new medical diagnostic tools with the primary ability to produce sufficiently strong magnetic fields to reorient hydrogen atoms within the body area that is being viewed.*

Neurones - *the primary cells of the brain and the yet-to-be explained origin of human consciousness. Each of the billions of neurones in the brain is inter-connected with thousands of others by short, incoming nerve fibers called dendrites, and long out-going fibers called axons.*

Obstructive stroke - *a stroke secondary to blockage of an artery, usually resulting from a clot. The clotted material may be of red blood cell origin but is usually a ball of blood platelets and fibrin. It may block at its site of origin on a damaged arterial wall or break away and create a block further down the blood vessel.*

Pravastatin - *the generic name for Pravachol.*

Progesterone - *a sex hormone vital to the reproductive process, synthesized in the body from its parent substance, cholesterol. Although primarily active in women as an "anti-estrogen" responsible for menses, this substance also has a vital role in males.*

Rhabdomyolysis - *an advanced form of muscle cell inflammation so severe as to break down the cellular structure of the cells. The components of this cellular destruction enter the blood stream and travel to the kidneys, causing obstruction of the filtration mechanism and resulting in kidney "failure."*

Sclerotic - *tissue hardened and sometimes swollen by the infiltration and accumulation of connective tissue fibers and calcium salts.*

Simvastatin - *the generic name for Zocor.*

Spreading depression - *a condition of overwhelming chemical chaos within the brain resulting in the complete loss of function, in which the area of the brain involved seems to no longer exist. Ordinarily, the condition is self-limiting but, if sufficiently prolonged, death of the tissue results.*

Statin drugs - *drugs with the ability to inhibit the so-called HMG-CoA reductase enzyme, a natural blocking point in the biosynthesis of cholesterol.*

Synapse - *the junction sites connecting the outgoing fibers of one brain cell with the incoming fibers of another. Transmission across this complex connection is usually mediated by a variety of specialized chemicals such as serotonin and adrenaline, know as neurotransmitters.*

Synaptogenic factor - *a chemical vital to the formation and function of a synapse. Recently this substance has been found to be cholesterol. The "housekeeper" cells of the brain, known as glial cells, that synthesize cholesterol as it is needed.*

Thalamic - *of or referring to the thalamus, a large mass of gray matter located deep within the brain that relays sensory stimuli to the cerebral cortex.*

Thrombophlebitis - *inflammation of the veins so severe as to cause clotting of the blood within. As these fragile masses of red blood cells break away from the parent clot and enter the venous circulation, they become a frequent source of blood clots to the lungs.*

Triglycerides - *one of the many forms of lipids in the body that result from the digestion of foodstuffs. Strangely enough, triglycerides result from the metabolism of carbohydrates.*

Ubiquinones - *a class of chemicals absolutely vital to energy production and membrane integrity of cells. In one form they work with the tiny powerhouses of energy within our cells known as mitochondria. In another form they help maintain the double-layered wall surrounding every cell in our body.*

Valsalva maneuver - *forced exhalation against a partially closed windpipe (glottis). This procedure causes predictable alterations in the blood flow through the various blood vessels within the chest cavity and restricts the return of blood from the lower half of the body. Monitoring the heart rate and blood pressure response during this procedure gives the examiner much information. In high performance flying, as in aerobatics, this procedure can also greatly increase tolerance to the pull of gravity.*

Vasodilator - *the ability to dilate or expand a blood vessel, enhancing blood flow.*

Vasospasm - *a contraction of the blood vessel which greatly narrows its size and restricts blood flow.*

Acetocholine

Boston Brain Science

Sharp PS

Adaptogen
Bacognize 150mg twice daily
Bacopa Cerebra

CPSIA information can be obtained
at www.ICGtesting.com
Printed in the USA
BVHW071603160721
612130BV00002B/90

9 781424 301621